Unraveling Dementia

Understanding and Beating Cognitive Decline

The Latest Science on Boosting Your Brain
and Thriving in Early-Stage Dementia

Cecile Black

For Mom,

with regret for what we didn't know

with hope that this book will help others do better.

Contents

Why I Wrote This Book

*It is not how much you do
but how much love you put in the doing.*

— Mother
Teresa

Some years ago I moved to another country, not considering the future of my aging parents who were fit and healthy at the time, and had my sister and niece living nearby.

Mom later had a mini stroke. Her doctors offered no indication about the possibility of dementia, and as she was already prone to forgetfulness, we didn't dwell on her occasional memory lapses.

Then, after a major blow when my sister and father passed away, there was a further decline in my mother's health and more mini strokes.

We noticed more forgetfulness and subtle behavioral changes, but not knowing anything factual about dementia and believing it was all about memory loss, we thought my mother's symptoms were down to grief and aging. She still recognized us and remembered events and conversations – that doesn't sound like dementia - right?

So, with no advice offered by doctors we did our best to assist my fiercely independent mother as much as we could. She agreed, eventually, to move closer to town into a small apartment with caretaking services and emergency-assistive technology and nearer to her granddaughter.

Over time, she changed, becoming angry and hurtful towards her family, exhibiting emotional outbursts, paranoia, confusion managing finances and money, and forgetfulness of everyday tasks like recipes she knew by heart. One night, she fell asleep with a pan on the stove, triggering building alarms that summoned police officers and firefighters and needing my niece to respond in the early hours.

While I was 10,000 km away, my niece, working full-time with a family including a disabled child, cared for my mother. I frequently traveled back and forth to assist where I could and eventually organized some basic in-home care.

A whirlwind of frustration, resentment, anger, guilt, sadness, and hopelessness swirled within us – emotions all tangled up with our deep love for her. It seemed as if nothing we did was good enough; even well-meaning church ladies who visited her experienced this new bitter, angry side; a once-kind woman transformed into someone mean, selfish, and demanding. It is hard to admit, but empathy and compassion were sometimes in short supply.

Then, one day, I got a call that she was in hospital with sepsis caused by a urinary tract infection that she had ignored and not told anyone about.

I spent two weeks at her bedside, witnessing my once amiable mother transformed dramatically; throwing objects and hot drinks at nurses, cursing angrily using words I didn't think she knew, and accusing everyone of trying to kill her. However, amid these painful episodes were moments when fear consumed her – not wanting to be alone in unfamiliar surroundings with strangers - begging to go home.

During the nights, I comforted her when she woke up startled and afraid. Her face would relax as she recognized me before falling back to sleep. One night will always stay with me; when she woke up, she looked at me with her beautiful blue eyes, clear and lucid; she smiled softly and said, "I love you...". At that moment, I had my mom back for one last time.

When advised the sepsis was too strong, and medication was not working, I wanted her to feel safe and comfortable, so I organized home hospice care, complete with a hospital bed and nursing staff. Content to return home, she passed away peacefully the next day.

Enduring my mother's decade-long health deterioration was emotionally draining for my family. The guilt of not being there enough and the anxiety from her increasingly bitter phone calls amplified my emotional distress. My niece and her husband would visit daily but often bore the brunt of my mother's complaints about their perceived indifference.

I only wish we had known more about dementia risks, causes, symptoms, and complications and could have learned more about the disease and how to manage it.

My memories of the precious moments will always outweigh the painful ones, but I do wish we had been better prepared at the start of her illness, and perhaps she could have enjoyed more happy moments with us all.

Could I have done more? Could I have been more understanding and possibly kinder? Could my mother and the family have worked together in earlier stages to implement strategies for better management and treatment? And most of all, if aware of potential health risks, could it have prevented the sepsis that ended her life? These questions linger, but I hope this book will illuminate such challenges for others.

This book provides valuable insights and strategies that can aid in slowing cognitive decline, maintaining independence and well-being, and ultimately continuing to create moments of happiness and joy in your life even as you move forward on the dementia journey.

Introduction

Dementia is a daunting word that can evoke fear in anyone who hears it. It is like a thief slowly stealing your most treasured possessions - memories and independence.

As someone who has experienced the hurt of seeing my mother as the disease changed her, slowly chipping away from the edges of her being, I wrote this book as a guide to what I wish my mother, and I had known right from the start. Had she been correctly diagnosed earlier, and if we had been empowered with this information, there is no telling what a difference this might have made.

But this is not a book about lamentation; it is a book of hope.

Hope for you, diagnosed with early-stage dementia, and your family. Hope for anyone worried about their own cognitive decline or that of someone they care about.

Having early-stage dementia is not the end, and with the correct information, you can plan and prepare for the future while taking steps to manage the progression and learning to thrive.

Together, we will embark on a journey to shed light on this condition, provide you with practical tools and strategies to navigate its winding paths, and guide you to living your best life while that thief peeps from around the corner.

Imagine standing before a curtain, behind which lies a world filled with uncertainty and fear - a world named dementia. As we pull back this curtain together, we will unveil truths about what lies ahead and how best to face these challenges head-on.

This book is structured like an unfolding story, your story, where each chapter delves deeper into different aspects of early-stage dementia. We will cover recognizing signs and symptoms, dealing with the diagnosis, making lifestyle changes to slow progression, and understanding how dementia evolves.

We will explore emotional support strategies for patients and caregivers because no one should face this journey alone. We will delve into coping mechanisms to make day-to-day living more accessible and ways in which joy can still be found amidst adversity.

Fear, anxiety, and depression are all part of this journey. Still, they do not define you or your loved ones' experience with dementia. Together, we will learn how best to cope with these emotions without being consumed by them. Finally, we will look towards the future. Although today may seem overwhelming, there is always tomorrow - a tomorrow that can be planned for and made brighter despite everything else going on around you.

The Uninvited Guest

You may not control all the events that happen to you,
but you can decide not to be reduced by them.

— Maya Angelou

When Marjorie, a retired schoolteacher, began forgetting familiar names and misplacing her glasses more frequently than usual, her children initially dismissed it as a byproduct of aging. However, they knew something was amiss when she started facing difficulties with tasks that once seemed second nature - like driving to the local grocery store or managing her finances.

A visit to the neurologist confirmed their fears: Marjorie had early-stage Alzheimer's disease. Shocked yet determined, her family vowed to support Marjorie through this journey. They delved into understanding dementia and its nuances, learning about its causes, risk factors, symptoms, and treatments.

Just like Marjorie's family, navigating through the early stages of dementia can be daunting for anyone. This book will guide you in understanding the various aspects of this condition and how to cope with them.

From early to the final stages of the disease, it impacts life in several ways:

Memory Loss

Dementia plays a critical role in memory loss and cognitive decline. This can be as simple as forgetting a name or misplacing your keys. However, it can also disrupt complex tasks like managing finances or following a recipe. For instance, you may need help remembering the steps of a dish you have cooked for years. However, don't lose heart; simple aids like reminder notes, alarms, or even digital apps can help manage these challenges.

Communication

You might struggle to find the right words or lose track of a conversation. This can be frustrating, but adopting strategies such as speaking slowly, using gestures, and maintaining eye contact can significantly improve communication. A fascinating study (Ashenden, 2020) showed that non-verbal communication could convey up to 93% of our messages, demonstrating that words are not everything.

Independence

Cognitive decline often impacts daily activities and independence. Tasks like dressing or cooking might become more complex.

However, breaking these tasks into smaller steps or using assistive devices can help maintain independence. For example, using a pill organizer can simplify medication management.

Unearthing Dementia's Causes and Risk Factors

Dementia isn't merely a part of aging; it is the result of diseases, including Alzheimer's, that affect the brain.

Risk factors vary from genetics to lifestyle choices. A study published in The Lancet (See, et al., 2023) identified twelve modifiable risk factors: less education in early life, hypertension in midlife, obesity after midlife, smoking, and diabetes. Managing these factors together can delay or prevent 40% of dementias.

Early Signs of Dementia: Beyond Memory Loss

Memory loss might be the most recognized symptom, but dementia encompasses more than just forgetfulness. It also affects cognitive abilities such as language, visual perception, and problem-solving skills.

Early signs include struggling with everyday tasks like cooking or cleaning, problems with language, mood changes, confusion about time and place, difficulty following conversations or TV shows, and repeating questions or stories within a short period.

Receiving a diagnosis of dementia can cause a whirlwind of emotions for both the person diagnosed and their loved ones - shock, disbelief, and fear followed by grief over the anticipated losses.

These feelings are normal reactions to an uncertain future but early-stage dementia is not the end and there is still joy to be found in life even after this diagnosis – albeit different from what you may have expected.

It is essential to take one step at a time. Seek support from friends and family members who understand your situation, join support groups to share experiences, and learn from others going through similar journeys.

Preparing For the Journey Ahead

There is currently no cure for dementia, but effective treatments can slow down its progression and improve quality of life significantly, particularly if started in the early stages when they are typically most effective.

Navigating through early-stage dementia requires understanding, acceptance, and preparation. Your path might not be easy, but with knowledge and determination, you will be better equipped to face what the future holds.

Know that you're not alone. Reach out to professionals who specialize in memory care and lean on supportive networks. Understand, prepare, like Marjorie who continues to live a fulfilling life surrounded by love and support despite her diagnosis. You, too, can do the same.

2

Dementia - Comprehensive Overview

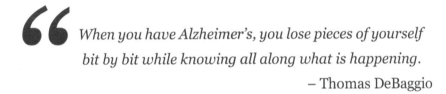 *When you have Alzheimer's, you lose pieces of yourself bit by bit while knowing all along what is happening.*
— Thomas DeBaggio

Dementia. A term that conjures up images of fading memories, lost conversations, and confusion. It's like a vast ocean where familiar shorelines slowly recede into the distance, leaving you adrift in a sea of forgetfulness. But what exactly is it?

Defining and Understanding Dementia

Dementia is not one specific disease but rather a term used to describe a group of symptoms associated with loss of memory or other cognitive skills severe enough to *reduce a person's ability to perform everyday activities*. It's like the sun setting on cognitive skills, clouding judgment, and blurring recognition.

Let's delve deeper into our understanding by visualizing brain cells as tiny cities with interconnected information highways.

In a healthy brain, cells interact harmoniously, allowing communication between different parts of the brain. In someone with dementia, however, this communication gets disrupted due to damage to these 'cities.' This could be compared to roads being blocked or telephone lines being cut off - gradually isolating cells until they can no longer function properly, leading to eventual shut down and resulting in chaos and disorder.

If you're worried about such symptoms persisting over time, consider consulting medical help promptly because when it comes to slowing down the progression, every second counts! And remember, sometimes it may just be stress or depression mimicking symptoms, so don't panic prematurely!

So, how do we tackle this abyss? There is no magic elixir yet, but specific lifestyle changes like regular exercise and maintaining social engagement can help slow down progression, much like watering plants regularly keeps them flourishing longer, even under harsh sunlight.

Lifestyle choices are crucial not just for those at risk of dementia but for everyone else too: eating healthily, keeping your mind and body active, and maintaining a positive attitude are essential to living and aging well.

Early detection of potential symptoms and prompt diagnosis matters. It can slow down progression with timely, proven intervention strategies like the ones described in this book.

Knowledge empowers us against our battles, so let this book serve as a step in your journey towards understanding and living with dementia effectively.

Common Dementia Misconceptions

Many misconceptions and myths surround dementia, especially in its early stages. These misunderstandings often lead to fear, stigma, and unnecessary distress for the person diagnosed and their loved ones. We debunk these myths and shed light on the reality of living with early-stage dementia.

Myth #1: Dementia is part of aging: Scientific research has shown that dementia is not a normal part of aging, contrary to what many people believe. This misconception often leads to delayed diagnosis and treatment, which can worsen the condition.

Myth #2: Dementia only affects older adults: Studies have found that dementia doesn't only affect older adults. While age does increase the risk factor for developing this disease, Early-onset Alzheimer's disease is a form of dementia that can occur in people as young as 30 or 40.

Myth #3: Memory loss equals dementia: Another common misconception about dementia is that it's solely characterized by memory loss. While this symptom is prevalent in most cases of Alzheimer's disease – the most common type of dementia – there are other forms where memory loss isn't the primary symptom.

Dementia involves difficulties with multiple areas of cognitive functioning, such as language skills, problem-solving abilities, or changes in personality and behavior. Factors like stress or depression can cause memory loss; it doesn't always signify dementia.

Myth #4: Alzheimer's and dementia are all the same: Alzheimer's disease is just one form among several types, including Vascular Dementia or Lewy Body Dementia. While they can share much in common, they are not all the same, and understanding the form and specific symptoms is an essential part of diagnosis, treatment, and living with the diseases.

Myth #5: Dementia diagnosis means life is over: A crucial point to remember is that being diagnosed with early-stage dementia doesn't mean your life ends here; instead, it marks a new chapter where adjustments need to be made.

Causes and Risk Factors

As we move through life, we all navigate a winding path. Sometimes, the road is smooth; other times, it's rocky; sometimes, it's sunny; other times stormy. But no matter what obstacles come our way, knowledge is always our most potent tool. In this section, we'll explore the causes and risk factors of early-stage dementia.

"Genes load the gun; lifestyle pulls the trigger."

- Dr Francis Collins

The Director of the National Institutes of Health expresses an undeniable truth in the above quote, perfectly capturing how genetics and lifestyle influence diseases like dementia.

Rare Genetic Conditions

Firstly, let's discuss genetics - one of those loaded guns. Some forms of dementia are entirely genetic – caused by specific gene mutations inherited from parents. Early-onset Alzheimer's Disease (EOAD), which affects people under 65, often falls into this category. However, these purely genetic cases are rare.

Genetic Risks Factors

More commonly seen are 'risk genes' that increase someone's likelihood but don't guarantee they will develop dementia. The most well-known is called ApoE4; if you inherit one copy from your parents, your Alzheimer's risk triples - inherit two copies, and it increases twelve-fold!

Sounds scary? Well, here's an 'ah-ha' moment, having a risk gene doesn't mean you'll get dementia; many ApoE4 carriers live long lives without developing symptoms.

Lifestyle Risk Factors

Now, let's move on to lifestyle factors - pulling that metaphorical trigger. Imagine them like buttons on a remote control – pressing some can reduce disease-risk volume while others can lower it.

Smoking? Volume goes up! High blood pressure or diabetes? Up again! Lack of exercise or unhealthy diet? You guessed it... up!

On the flip side, though - brain-healthy foods like fruits and vegetables? Volume goes down! Regular physical activity, especially in midlife? Down again! Maintaining strong social connections and mental stimulation throughout life also play their part in reducing risk volume.

One critical enemy to watch out for is chronic stress. Research suggests prolonged stress may damage brain areas key to memory.

> *Genes increase the risk of early-stage dementia, but lifestyle choices significantly determine whether these genetic risks become a reality.*

Consider that even among identical twins (who share all the same genes), when one twin develops Alzheimer's during their lifetime, only about half their siblings do too, suggesting environmental factors substantially impact disease development.

So, how do we act armed with this knowledge?

Lifestyle Choices to Manage Risk Factors

According to Alzheimer's Association (2021) (Alzheimer Association, 2021), nearly 6 million Americans live with Alzheimer's. As the older population expands, this will rise alarmingly by almost threefold by mid-century unless we find ways to slow its progression effectively.

Tips to Manage Risk Factors

- **Understand Your Genetic Risk:** If there's a family history of early-onset Alzheimer's, consider speaking with a genetic counselor who can help interpret any potential risks associated with your health picture.
- **Adopt A Brain-Healthy Lifestyle:** Incorporate regular exercise into your routine; adopt a balanced nutritious diet; quit smoking.
- **Manage Chronic Conditions:** Keep tabs on high blood pressure or diabetes if present.
- **Reduce Stress**: Practice relaxation techniques, meditation or yoga.
- **Stay Socially and Mentally Engaged:** Keep learning new things; maintain active social ties.

In conclusion:

- Dementia isn't simply about 'bad' genes but rather an interaction between genes and the environment.
- Knowing your risk allows appropriate actions toward prevention.
- Managing modifiable risk factors provides your best defense against onset and progression.

The Different Faces of Dementia

Most people associate dementia with Alzheimer's Disease not knowing that there are several types, each with its own characteristics and effects on cognitive function. Sadly, as my experience with my mother demonstrated, being unaware of these different presentations can lead to assumptions, dismissing symptoms, and cognitive decline freely progressing when early diagnosis and treatment might have slowed or prevented it.

DIFFERENT TYPES OF DEMENTIA

ALZHEIMER'S DISEASE
Most Common 60% - 80% of cases
Initial signs - forget recent events or conversations .Advances to disorientation, behavior changes, memory loss Can impact physical capabilities like walking or swallowing

VASCULAR DEMENTIA
5% -10% of cases
Reduced blood flow damages to brain cells. After stroke or ministrokes. Symptoms vary based on affected brain region Difficulty with problem-solving, focus, or slowed thinking.

LEWY BODY DEMENTIA
5% 10% of cases
Abnormal protein deposits in nerve cells. Problems with thinking, behavior, mood, and movement Symptoms may fluctuate throughout the day

FRONTO - TEMPORAL
5% - 10% of cases
Damage to the frontal lobes of the brain. Can show poor judgment or impulse control Difficulty making decisions and complex thinking

OTHER
5% - 10% combined
Symptoms caused by conditions - Huntingdon's, Parkinson's, Alcohol related, Down syndrome, HIV

MIXED
Symptoms combined. from more than one source. Not attributed to a single cause; results. from a combination of factors

EARLY ONSET
5% - 10% combined
Affects under 65's
Presents differently Behavioral changes; difficulty with vision/ language. Harder to diagnose Progresses more rapidly

The Seven Stages of Dementia

Understanding how dementia progresses allows you to recognize its initial signs and seek medical advice as early as possible. It prepares us better to manage its subsequent stages effectively while providing emotional support for those affected during this challenging period.

NO IMPAIRMENT

No obvious signs exhibited.

MILD COGNITIVE DECLINE

Losing track of familiar objects
Forgetting names of friends and family.

EARLY-STAGE

Forget appointments; lose items; forget words; repeat things; may get lost. Difficulty with organization, focus and complex tasks; poorer functioning at work

MODERATE 4

Behavior change, moods, withdrawn and unresponsive; may be in denial of symptoms

Struggle with everyday activities; forget recent events

MODERATELY SEVERE 5

Unable to carry out daily activities. Confusion, disorientation, insomnia, wandering. Emotional and aggressive. Mental decline and difficulty problem-solving

SEVERE 6

Need full-time care
Urinary or faecal incontinence
Aggression, anxiety. Paranoia or delusions. May not recognize family members

VERY SEVERE 7

Unable to speak
Difficulty with movement and coordination, chewing/ swallowing

Unmasking the Early Signs of Dementia

Our brains are like vast, intricate tapestries woven with threads of memories, thoughts, and emotions. They narrate our past, shape our present, and influence our future. But what happens when those threads start to fray?

More than just forgetfulness or occasional confusion; dementia is a syndrome characterized by memory loss and a decline in cognitive abilities severe enough to interfere with daily life. Its onset might seem insidious, often mistaken for typical aging signs rather than the initiation of a disease process. However, knowing these nuances could be your most potent weapon against dementia.

Several recent studies (Johansson, et al., 2019), (Lanctôt, et al., 2017) have found that noticeable shifts in behavior, such as increased agitation, anxiety, or apathy, could be early signs of dementia. These symptoms often precede memory loss and cognitive decline, typically associated with this disease. If you are trying to identify potential signs within yourself or a loved one at home, follow these five steps.

Agitation, anxiety, or apathy often precede memory loss and cognitive decline.

Tips for Detecting Potential Symptoms

1. **Be observant** of routine behavior patterns.
2. **Keep track** and note if you notice consistent disruptions due to memory issues, including frequency and severity.
3. **Consult professionals** - don't hesitate to seek professional help if unsure.
4. **Keep calm** and learn about dementia and its management strategies.
5. **Stay healthy** - adopt lifestyle modifications promoting brain health.

Signs and Symptoms of Early-Stage Dementia

Scientists have identified symptoms associated with early-stage dementia. These include but are not limited to:

- trouble remembering names or recent events, losing items, and being unable to retrace steps
- difficulty with familiar tasks, especially complex ones like managing finances
- challenges with planning or solving problems
- confusion with time or place
- behavior changes - increased agitation, anxiety, or apathy
- difficulty understanding images, problems speaking or writing words
- decreased or poor judgment
- withdrawal from work or social activities

For cases exhibiting severe symptoms rapidly over weeks or months instead of years (Rapidly Progressive Dementia), seek immediate medical attention – it may be potentially reversible if diagnosed promptly.

Studies testing thousands of people for early-stage symptoms over several years provide convincing evidence that such changes are possible indicators of an underlying disease process. In early-stage dementia, a person may still be able to function independently but have trouble remembering names or recent events. They might also experience mood swings and increased anxiety.

Onset of Early-Stage Dementia: Margaret's Story

Friends started noticing something different about Margaret. Her usual cheerful demeanor seemed slightly subdued. Her laughter didn't ring out quite as often or as loud. And then there were moments when she'd pause mid-conversation, looking lost and confused before snapping back to reality.

It was so subtle initially that most people dismissed it as mere signs of aging. But over time, these changes became more pronounced.

One incident vividly stood out: at a charity event organized by her community church. Margaret managed the raffle tickets but struggled to track sold and unsold ones that day. People started whispering about how strange it was that Margaret couldn't seem to handle something she had done so quickly countless times before.

The whispers grew louder when Margaret began forgetting the names of people, even those she had known for decades. Struggling to recall who they were until someone gently, or not so sometimes, jogged her memory.

Margaret's story serves as a reminder that even seemingly insignificant changes in behavior could indicate something much more severe lurking underneath. It underlines why we need greater awareness about early-stage dementia - recognizing its symptoms and understanding its progression over time.

Why Early Detection and Diagnosis Matters

A study published in 'The Lancet' highlighted that diagnosing dementia early allows for timely therapeutic interventions that can slow down disease progression significantly (Livingston et al., 2020). So, if any symptoms feel alarmingly persistent or progressive - don't ignore them! You should consult a healthcare professional for further evaluation.

Early recognition of dementia symptoms leads to timely diagnosis and intervention, which can slow disease progression.

However, diagnosing dementia isn't like to assembling a jigsaw puzzle; all pieces fitting together perfectly are not required for accurate identification. Instead, think of it as painting a picture where each symptom adds color and depth, leading toward an overall diagnosis.

Mary was a retired schoolteacher from Boston; she started noticing difficulty remembering names and appointments when she was around 65. Initially dismissing it as part of growing old, her concerns grew when she began forgetting conversations she'd had just a few hours before – prompting her to visit a neurologist who diagnosed her with early-stage Alzheimer's disease. Acknowledging these symptoms enabled an early diagnosis, allowing better management strategies - lifestyle modifications like diet changes and regular physical exercise paired with prescribed medication helped slow her disease progression considerably.

Roadblocks to Early Detection and Diagnosis

Initially, Margaret dismissed symptoms as a normal part of aging. But on noticing other changes, she immediately took action to get a health check. It is easy to ignore red flags as 'just getting old,' but if in any doubt, check out concerns with your doctor. The earlier you do this, you can either put your mind at rest that all is well, or if early dementia is detected, immediately take action to arrest further decline.

A major roadblock for some people is fear. Getting lost in anxiety-ridden what-ifs only lets valuable time slip away leaving symptoms to worsen.

Dementia is like an iceberg; what we see on the surface is only a fraction of what's underneath. Initial signs might seem trivial but just as an iceberg can cause drastic consequences if underestimated (think Titanic), ignoring early signs of dementia can lead to severe consequences, too.

> *Recognizing symptoms and seeking medical advice early helps manage the disease and provides valuable time to prepare for what lies ahead. An early diagnosis also allows participation in clinical trials with access to new treatments before they're widely available.*

If you are experiencing any signs of cognitive decline, seek medical advice promptly for an accurate diagnosis.

Potential Dementia Complications

As a chronic disorder caused by brain disease or injury, dementia is often associated with various complications.

According to research (Iaboni, Phil, & Flint, 2013), people with dementia are at an increased risk of developing physical and psychological complications such as falls, depression, and anxiety.

Therefore, it becomes crucial to understand these potential complications to provide appropriate support as the disease progresses.

1. **Reduce the risk of falls** through regular physical activity to help improve mood and maintain balance and coordination.
2. **Reduce feelings of isolation** and depression by maintaining social interactions.
3. **Prevent accidents** by providing a safe environment at home by removing tripping hazards and installing safety measures in bathrooms and kitchens.

4. **Detect changes as early as possible** with regular check-ups by healthcare professionals to identify any new symptoms or changes in behavior that might indicate disease progression.

Overcoming Dementia Stigma

While making a recent BBC UK documentary program[1] that followed the progress of people coping with dementia, one message came across clearly: that a diagnosis of dementia is not the end. For a condition still so stigmatized as dementia, that is ground-breaking.

In the late 1970s, Glenn Campbell, a renowned country singer, was at the peak of his career. His songs were topping the charts, and he was on tour worldwide. But as the years rolled by, something seemed off. He would forget lyrics to songs he had sung hundreds of times before; he would lose track of conversations midway and sometimes even forget where he was.

It wasn't until 2011 that Glenn's family publicly announced that he had been diagnosed with Alzheimer's. Suddenly, it all made sense, but instead of retreating into silence or shame due to the societal stigma associated with dementia, Glenn did something extraordinary.

He decided to go public about his diagnosis. He embarked on a "Goodbye Tour," performing over 150 shows worldwide while battling Alzheimer's. The tour was documented in an award-winning

---

[1] How BBC Two's latest documentary 'Dementia and Us' captured the realities of dementia, 2021

film called "I'll Be Me", offering viewers an intimate look into Glenn's struggle with dementia.

The truth is that dementia is still stigmatized in our society today. People with this condition are often marginalized or treated differently because others may not fully understand what they're going through.

A study published by Batsch & Mittelman (World Alzheimer Report 2012 Overcoming the stigma of dementia, 2012) found that people living with dementia often feel excluded from everyday life activities and social interactions due to their cognitive impairments coupled with societal misunderstandings about their condition.

But just like Glenn Campbell demonstrated so bravely through his Goodbye Tour – there are ways to combat this stigma surrounding dementia.

Education– understanding what dementia is and how it affects individuals can help reduce misconceptions about it. This involves educating ourselves and those around us, including children who may struggle to comprehend why grandma or grandpa no longer remembers them.

Empathy – putting ourselves in the shoes of someone with dementia can help us better understand their struggles and treat them more compassionately rather than out casting them because they're different now.

Open conversations – When individuals share their experiences openly without fear or shame, it normalizes the condition and breaks down barriers created by stigmatization.

Positive portrayals of people living with dementia – this can challenge negative stereotypes. Highlighting their abilities rather than focusing on impairments fosters an environment where they are seen as valuable members of society who can contribute meaningfully despite their diagnosis.

Advocate – local and national policy changes that ensure inclusivity for people suffering from such cognitive disorders could make all the difference!

The fear, misunderstanding, and negative attitudes surrounding dementia often leads to social isolation, loneliness, and depression. So, let's take inspiration from brave souls like Glenn Campbell, who chose not only to face their battles head-on but also shine light upon dementia, which need our understanding rather than our judgment.

Summing Up

Getting a diagnosis of dementia is a significant blow, likely leaving you reeling from shock, disbelief, fear, and emotional overwhelm. While you process these emotions, reach out for professional support and let the reality of the situation sink in.

Early diagnosis and timely interventions can slow down progression and enable you to live better for longer and you can enjoy more time with the people you love as you look for new advances and research that may delay progression even more.

Key Takeaways

- *The World Health Organisation estimates around 50 million people worldwide have dementia.*
- *Dementia represents multiple conditions marked by progressive cognitive impairments.*
- *Damage caused interrupts communications within brain cells, significantly hampering functionality.*
- *Age isn't the sole risk factor; genetics plays a significant role, too.*
- *The first step towards fighting dementia begins by recognizing these symptoms early on. Regularly use self-evaluations to aid identification.*
- *Know the common early-stage dementia - symptoms go beyond typical age-related forgetfulness and impact daily life noticeably,*
- *Overcome fears preventing you from seeking help - diagnosis at the earliest possible stage aids management strategies tremendously.*
- *Memory loss, on its own, does not indicate dementia. Significant memory loss affecting daily routines isn't normal aging!*

3

Navigating the Fog

 Courage doesn't always roar...
sometimes courage is the quiet voice at the end of the day
saying... I will try again tomorrow.
— Mary Anne Radmacher

Like a ship sailing into a foggy morning, the onset of early-stage dementia can often feel like you're moving into an unknown world, but it's not an insurmountable obstacle. A boat has its compass and maps to navigate the misty waters, just as with the right strategies and tools you can still find your way.

Living with early-stage dementia doesn't mean the end of a meaningful life. Instead, it's a new journey that requires rediscovering strengths, adapting to changes, and using every tool at your disposal. Like that ship sailing into the foggy morning, you might not see what's ahead clearly. Still, you can navigate your way forward with resilience and grace.

From Shock to Acceptance: Coping After a Dementia Diagnosis

The moment the word 'dementia' escapes from the lips of your doctor, you might feel as if the ground has been swept away beneath your feet. A rush of emotions engulfs you and leaves you gasping for air. Fear about what lies in store, anger at why it happened, sadness at the perceived loss of identity or independence, guilt over potential burdens placed on loved ones.

I want you to know that every feeling you experience is valid. It's okay to grieve for what was while learning how to embrace what will be.

Unraveling dementia begins by accepting its presence in your life. This acceptance isn't about giving up or surrendering but adapting to this new reality to best navigate it.

> *"Acceptance is not about giving up or surrendering, but rather acknowledging the reality of your situation and choosing to live life as fully as possible despite it."*
>
> *- Unknown*

Acceptance doesn't mean resignation; it means understanding that something is what it is and there's got to be a way through it, paving the way towards resilience and changing your lifestyle and habits to manage the disease and hopefully slow down progression.

A research study published in The American Journal of Geriatric Psychiatry found evidence suggesting individuals who accepted their diagnosis reported improved mental health outcomes than those who did not (Rüegger-Frey et al., 2017). This indicates acceptance can potentially pave the way towards resilience.

Consider Jane's story: A vibrant woman diagnosed with early-stage dementia at age 55 who refused to let her condition define her fate. Instead, she embraced her situation as a challenge rather than an obstacle. She started journaling her daily experiences as a therapeutic outlet. She became an advocate for early detection among friends and community groups.

Your power lies in your resilience and strength to face adversity, transforming echoes of despair into songs of hope.

One solution gaining popularity among cognitive experts involves Cognitive Behavioral Therapy (CBT) to manage distress associated with dementia diagnosis (Sadowsky & Galvin, 2012). CBT challenges negative thought patterns and helps individuals develop effective coping strategies.

In another case study highlighted in the Aging & Mental Health Journal (Kiosses et al., 2015), George, a retired engineer diagnosed with mild cognitive impairment, showed reduced anxiety levels after undergoing an eight-week Cognitive Behavioral Therapy (CBT) program designed for people with similar diagnoses.

Remember that your journey is unique and individual. Every person's experience is different. No right or wrong ways exist to feel or cope with the situation.

Understanding Your Feelings

Feelings of shock, denial, anxiety, and sadness are common reactions after a dementia diagnosis. It's essential to acknowledge these feelings instead of suppressing them. Remember that there's no right or wrong way to respond - everyone copes differently.

Experts from the Mayo Clinic suggest that "talking about your feelings can often help relieve some stress and help you gain perspective."

By acknowledging your feelings, utilizing available resources, participating in self-care activities, and planning proactively you will find your way.

If you implement the practical advice outlined in this book, you will be better prepared emotionally and armed with supportive coping strategies ranging from practical approaches, such as maintaining a daily routine and using reminders for tasks, to more therapeutic methods, like engaging in physical activities and hobbies that stimulate mental activity.

For instance, regular exercise helps maintain good blood flow to the brain and may encourage new brain cell growth. Hobbies or pastimes you enjoy can distract from negative emotions while keeping your mind active.

In 2018, researchers at University College London (Socially active 60-year-olds face lower dementia risk, 2019) published a study indicating that social interaction could significantly slow down the decline in patients who have dementia. Participants involved in group activities displayed slower cognitive decline than those who did not regularly participate in social interactions.

Tips to Process Emotions Following Diagnosis

- Remember that you are more than just your diagnosis.
- Allow yourself time to process any feelings.
- Reach out to professional therapists and counselors to help you deal with the emotional impact of such a diagnosis.
- Find therapeutic outlets like journaling or painting.
- Join support groups where others share similar experiences.
- Practice mindfulness techniques like meditation or yoga.

Coping Strategies for People with Early-Stage Dementia and Their Families

In a study published in the International Journal of Geriatric Psychiatry (Aguirre, et al., 2012), strategies such as cognitive stimulation therapy (CST), which involves engaging in mentally stimulating activities, and person-centred care (PCC), which focuses on individual needs and preferences, have shown promising results.

The study found that people with dementia who participated in CST sessions significantly improved their cognitive function and quality of life. Similarly, PCC reduced agitation and improved social interaction.

This suggests that instead of relying solely on medication, incorporating these non-drug approaches into your care plan can lead to better outcomes.

Maintaining an active lifestyle can significantly contribute to managing symptoms of dementia. Regular exercise improves physical health and positively affects mood and sleep patterns.

Cognitive stimulation activities such as puzzles or memory games can help slow cognitive decline while providing a constructive outlet for stress relief.

Additional tips include establishing calming routines before bedtime if sleep disturbance becomes an issue or seeking professional help if depression seems likely.

More information on strategies to help manage symptoms and slow the progression of dementia is provided in later chapters of this book.

Tips for Coping After Diagnosis

- Acknowledge your feelings regarding the diagnosis.
- Begin working on acceptance.
- Establish practical daily routines.
- Engage regularly in physical activity.
- Seek social interactions.
- Consult professionals when necessary.

Caregiver Well-Being

Caregivers might experience various emotions, from frustration and guilt to loneliness and exhaustion. Seeking support groups or counseling services can provide much-needed emotional assistance.

A study by Stanford Medicine highlights the importance of caregiver self-care, stating that "caregivers' physical health often deteriorates due to neglecting their care when consumed by caregiving responsibilities.

This book includes a *caregiver guide* providing strategies for self-care and coping with challenges.

Maintaining Independence in Daily Activities

Scientific research indicates that following a consistent daily routine helps to maintain independence, improve quality of life, and slow disease progression.

According to a study published in the American Journal of Geriatric Psychiatry (Gitlin, et al., 2008), following a structured daily routine has reduced anxiety and agitation, improved sleep patterns, and improved quality of life. Routines provide structure and familiarity, which can help reduce confusion and stress in people with this condition.

Another study published in The Journal of Gerontology (DiPietro, 2001) found that people engaging in regular, structured physical activity are more likely to maintain their ability to perform daily tasks, including dressing, bathing, and cooking. This helps retain independence, boosting self-esteem and overall mental well-being.

It's highly recommended to establish a consistent daily routine tailored according to your preferences and abilities and adjust over time until finding the one that works best.

An ideal daily routine should include regular mealtimes, time for physical activities such as walking or gardening, rest, and cognitive stimulation activities like reading or puzzles.

When daily routines consistently incorporate these elements (even if it's challenging due to fluctuating moods or energy levels), you can experience enhanced mood, improved memory function, and prolonged autonomy.

This is a far cry from the feelings of helplessness that often accompany living with dementia. By prioritizing active physical and cognitive engagement, you're not just managing symptoms - you're actively improving your quality of life and maintaining capabilities and independence for longer.

"When people with dementia are empowered in ways that assure their continued growth and development, they can deal more effectively with their impairment."

- Daniel Kuhn

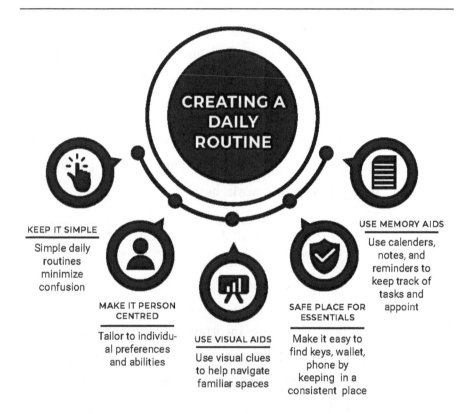

CREATING A DAILY ROUTINE

KEEP IT SIMPLE
Simple daily routines minimize confusion

MAKE IT PERSON CENTRED
Tailor to individual preferences and abilities

USE VISUAL AIDS
Use visual clues to help navigate familiar spaces

SAFE PLACE FOR ESSENTIALS
Make it easy to find keys, wallet, phone by keeping in a consistent place

USE MEMORY AIDS
Use calenders, notes, and reminders to keep track of tasks and appoint

A stable daily routine enriched with physical activity could be a strong ally for you and those when caring you. Not only does it offer comfort through predictability, but it also aids in preserving mental health.

Driving Safely and When to Stop

Early-stage dementia can impact your ability to drive safely. A study conducted by the American Academy of Neurology (D.J.Iverson, et al., 2010) found that drivers with mild dementia were more likely to be involved in car accidents compared to those without any cognitive impairment.

The research shows that while some people with early-stage dementia may still be able to drive, their risk of unsafe driving increases significantly as the disease progresses. This is due to various factors such as memory loss, difficulty concentrating, slower reaction times, and problems with spatial awareness.

Therefore, it's crucial for individuals diagnosed with early-stage dementia and their families to have open conversations about when it might be time to stop driving. Regular assessments by healthcare professionals can also help monitor changes in driving abilities over time.

While giving up driving can feel like a loss of independence, alternative transportation options such as public transit, ride-sharing services, or relying on family members and friends for rides are available.

Moreover, ceasing to drive does not mean ending one's social life or mobility. Studies show that planning for this transition can lead to a better quality of life in the long run by reducing anxiety around potential accidents and promoting safer environments for everyone on the road.

Traveling Safely

Traveling can be beneficial for individuals with early-stage dementia, as it can provide stimulation, enjoyment, and a break from routine. However, it also comes with its own set of challenges.

According to a study published in the Journal of Travel Medicine (Sadlon, Ensslin, Freystätter, Gagesch, & Heike A Bischoff-Ferrari, 2020), people with early-stage dementia who travel may experience disorientation and confusion due to environmental changes, which can cause stress and anxiety. Therefore, careful planning is crucial when traveling with this condition.

Tips for Travelling with Early-Stage Dementia

- **Always carry identification**, including name, contact information, and details about medical conditions. A study by the Alzheimer's Association suggests using a safe return program or GPS tracking device for added security.
- **Maintain familiar routines** as much as possible during travel. According to experts at the Mayo Clinic, sticking to regular eating and sleeping schedules can help reduce confusion in people with dementia.
- **Avoid overly crowded or noisy destinations** as these environments could cause distress. Go for quiet places which have a calming effect on the mind.
- **Always consult with your healthcare provider** before planning any trip. They can provide advice tailored your needs and health status.

With proper planning and precautions based on scientific research and expert advice, you can ensure a safe and enjoyable journey for everyone involved.

Navigating Holidays and Special Occasions

As we already know, maintaining familiar routines helps to reduce confusion and anxiety for people with dementia. This means that it's beneficial to keep traditions as similar as possible during holidays or special occasions. However, modifications may be necessary to accommodate changing abilities.

For instance, if a family tradition involves a complicated game or activity that could frustrate someone with cognitive impairment, replacing it with something simpler and more relaxing is better.

Similarly, large gatherings can sometimes overwhelm people with dementia; smaller or quieter celebrations may prove less stressful.

Another critical factor is the environment. Research from The Gerontologist suggests that well-lit spaces can improve mood and behavior in people with dementia. So, when planning holiday decorations or choosing venues for special occasions, consider how lighting might affect overall comfort and enjoyment.

Lastly, remember the importance of patience and understanding during these times. It might take longer to do certain things, or you may not remember everyone at the gathering, but this doesn't mean you aren't able to enjoy the experience.

In conclusion:

- Keep traditions consistent but flexible enough to adapt as needed.
- Create comfortable environments.
- Exercise patience and empathy.

These steps are scientifically backed in helping those with early-stage dementia navigate holidays and special occasions more comfortably.

Socializing and Community Involvement

> *"Laughter lets me relax; it reminds me that I can enjoy life despite dementia."*
>
> *- Norms McNamara*

Alice was a vibrant, energetic woman in her early 70s with a love for gardening and a knack for storytelling. She was always the life of the party until she was diagnosed with early-stage dementia.

Alice started to forget things. Not just where she left her keys or what she had for breakfast but essential dates like birthdays and anniversaries. It scared her. She withdrew from friends and family, fearing they would judge or pity her.

Her condition worsened rapidly within six months of self-isolation.

Contrast this with George, another lively septuagenarian diagnosed with early-stage dementia around the same time as Alice. George loved chess and jazz music. Like Alice, he too began forgetting things - his favorite songs, how to set up the chessboard.

But instead of withdrawing from society, George sought help from his local community center, which offered programs designed for people with cognitive decline.

George regularly attended these sessions where he interacted with others going through similar experiences. He participated in group activities that stimulated his mind – like simple board games and memory exercises involving music therapy.

Six months later, while Alice's condition had significantly deteriorated due to isolation, George's symptoms progressed much slower despite having the same diagnosis.

Why such a stark difference?

According to a study published in The Journal of Gerontology: Psychological Sciences (2019) (Broader social interaction keeps older adults more active, 2019), social engagement significantly positively affects cognitive functioning among older adults, including those suffering from dementia.

The researchers found that individuals who regularly engaged in social activities showed less cognitive decline than those who isolated themselves after being diagnosed with dementia.

So, here's what you can learn from Alice and George's stories: Having dementia is not an end-all-be-all situation if you don't let it be one!

Staying socially active could slow down cognitive decline associated with dementia. In contrast, isolation and loneliness have been linked to an increased risk of Alzheimer's disease (Akhter-Khan, et al., 2021)

While living with early-stage dementia may pose challenges, staying socially active could slow its progression while improving overall well-being.

Tips for Staying Connected

- Participate in local events or clubs.
- Keep in regular contact with friends and family members.
- Volunteer for a cause close to your heart.
- Join support groups designed for people dealing with similar conditions where they can share experiences and coping strategies.

Adjustments at Home for a Safe and Comfortable Sanctuary

The keys jingle, the door creaks open, you step inside, and it instantly feels like home. It's that comforting scent of familiarity, the sight of your favorite chair in its usual spot by the window, or perhaps the dog greeting you with a wagging tail. Now imagine this same sanctuary becoming confusing or even hazardous due to an ailment such as dementia.

As cognitive abilities decline because of dementia, so do spatial awareness and visual perception. A once familiar space can become challenging to navigate, but simple changes can make all the difference. A study published in The Gerontologist Journal (2013) (Sheffield, Smith, & Becker, 2013) found that environmental modifications significantly reduced behavioral symptoms for people living at home. Minor adjustments can help to maintain physical well-being and mental health.

Tips for Adjustments at Home

- Declutter the house regularly. Remove tripping hazards such as cables and wires running across the floor. Tape down or remove rugs to prevent trip hazards.
- Ensure clear pathways.
- Label household items clearly.
- Use contrasting colors.
- Install support rails where necessary.
- Prioritize good lighting, especially for night-time navigation.
- Seek professional help if conditions worsen despite precautions.
- Use creativity when implementing these adjustments. For example, use brightly colored sticky notes for labeling instead of plain ones – turning it into an engaging activity rather than a chore.

MAKING ADJUSTMENTS AT HOME

KITCHEN

Label cupboards or drawers - 'Spoons', 'Plates', etc., to aid recall.
Use contrasting colors - a red plate on a white tablecloth is easier to distinguish than a white on a white.

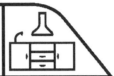

BATHROOM

Install grab bars near toilet and bath for added support and safety.
Ensure well-lit spaces, particularly at night; consider motion sensor lights for extra safety.

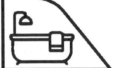

BEDROOM

Clear pathways to the bathroom and kitchen of tripping hazards to prevent falls
Use motion sensor lights for safety in case of nighttime wandering Position a lamp within easy reach when in bed

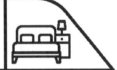

LIVING ROOM

Remove clutter to create a safe and accessible environment.
Choose round-edged furniture over sharp-edged to minimize injury from accidental bumps

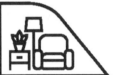

Suppose the condition worsens, causing you start to wander dangerously or fall frequently despite these precautions. In that case, professional advice should be sought immediately – either consult a doctor about possible medication alterations or consider installing surveillance cameras for constant monitoring during high-risk times like late nights.

Remember, every slight adjustment today creates a safer, more comfortable sanctuary. You can find many great tips this article at Bright Focus Foundation. (Allen, 2021).

Technical Tools for Daily Life

Technology such as smartphones and tablets are powerful tools in aiding individuals with early-stage dementia to maintain independence and cognitive abilities for extended periods.

As well as providing practical assistance, these tools also give you a sense of control over your life and reduce feelings of anxiety and depression often associated with the disease.

If you or a loved one has been diagnosed with this condition, consider user-friendly tech tools to assist in daily routines. There are numerous apps and tools designed specifically for people with dementia that can assist with everyday tasks like setting reminders for medication, keeping track of appointments, or even helping to navigate familiar routes.

Getting used to new technologies might take some time, so patience and support are crucial during this process. Still, it will be worth it for increased independence and mental agility.

How John Glenn Embraced Technology

John Glenn, the first American to orbit Earth and a long-time U.S. Senator, was no stranger to challenges. But when he was diagnosed with early-stage dementia in his late 80s, it presented a new obstacle.

John had always been an active man. He loved hiking in the woods near his home and spending time with his grandchildren. But as his memory started to fade, these activities became increasingly difficult. He'd forget where he put things or lose track of conversations halfway through.

His daughter noticed these changes and wanted to help her father maintain independence while ensuring his safety. She began researching technology tools designed for people with dementia.

One device she found was a GPS tracking system that could be worn like a wristwatch. This tool would allow John's family to locate him if he ever got lost during one of his hikes or walks around town - a common issue for some with dementia.

Another tool she discovered was an automated medication dispenser that would alert John when it was time for him to take his medicine - another critical task that often becomes challenging due to memory loss.

John's daughter also discovered several smartphone apps designed specifically for individuals with early-stage dementia.

These tools were game changers for John and gave him back some control over his life despite the disease's progression.

Most importantly, they provided peace of mind for John and those who cared about him deeply.

Technology can't cure dementia or reverse its effects. Still, it offers solutions that help preserve dignity and make daily life more manageable for those with the disease and their loved ones.

Preserving Dignity as Dementia Progresses

> *"I'm still me no matter how my days look."*
>
> *- unknown dementia patient*

Maintaining a sense of dignity is crucial for the well-being of individuals living with dementia. A study published in the Journal of Clinical Nursing has shown that despite cognitive decline, people with dementia can still perceive and experience feelings related to their dignity.

The study highlights that personal identity, autonomy, and relationships are vital to preserving dignity. The researchers found that when these aspects are respected and supported, it boosts self-esteem, and feelings of being valued.

Regular visits from family members or friends can provide emotional support and reinforce feelings of being loved and valued. Even if communication becomes difficult due to disease progression, simply being present can positively impact emotional well-being.

Bessie's Story

Bessie was an extraordinary woman. In her prime, she'd been a renowned physicist known for her ground-breaking research in quantum mechanics. Her mind was a treasure trove of knowledge, but more than that, it was the core of her identity.

Then dementia came knocking.

It started subtly - misplaced keys, forgotten appointments. But soon, it escalated to lost memories and confusion about familiar faces. Bessie's once vibrant world began to fade into a foggy haze.

Now imagine being Bessie's daughter, Emma. You've watched your mother's brilliance dimmed by this relentless disease. You've witnessed her struggle with simple tasks that she once did effortlessly.

But here's where things take an exciting turn. Despite the heartbreak and challenges, Emma found hope in preserving her mother's dignity.

She had read a study conducted by University College London (UCL), which revealed that personalized care could significantly improve the quality of life for people with dementia. This wasn't about finding a cure but making every day count.

Inspired by this research, Emma acted. She transformed their home into a sanctuary filled with reminders of Bessie's accomplishments and passions: framed certificates from physics conferences hung on walls, shelves adorned with favorite quantum mechanics books, and family photos scattered throughout rooms.

This approach worked wonders! Whenever Bessie became confused or agitated, these visual cues would often calm her down and sometimes even spark moments of clarity.

Emma also ensured Bessie remained socially engaged as much as possible within their community – frequent visits from friends who shared stories from their pasts and kept connections alive.

And so, they continued - not merely surviving but living each day to its fullest despite the circumstances.

The crux is not just about dealing with dementia; how you deal with it matters, too! It might seem like an uphill battle initially. Still, if you choose compassion over despair and proactive steps over resignation, you can take steps to maintain dignity– just like Emma did for Bessie.

Promoting Mental Health and Well Being

Living with early-stage dementia can be a time of uncertainty, fear, and confusion, but it's also an opportunity to take charge of your health and well-being, find new ways to connect with the world, and focus on what truly matters.

The first step is understanding that dementia is not just about memory loss; it affects every aspect of your life - emotional, physical, social, and spiritual.

Find comfort knowing you are not alone, and you can reach out for support from friends and family, medical professionals, therapists, support groups, and online communities. Connect with these networks when you need to for emotional support, health concerns, or to benefit from the shard experiences and insights of others in a similar situation.

Staying physically active with regular exercise or simple activities such as gardening and walking improves mood and energy levels while reducing anxiety and symptoms of depression.

Moreover, stimulating your mind by engaging in activities you enjoy – hobbies, reading books, solving puzzles, or playing games that challenge your cognitive abilities can help slow down the progression of dementia symptoms.

Last but most importantly, maintain open communication with your loved ones about how you feel emotionally. Emotional well-being is as crucial as physical health in managing early-stage dementia.

MENTAL AND PHYSICAL WELL-BEING

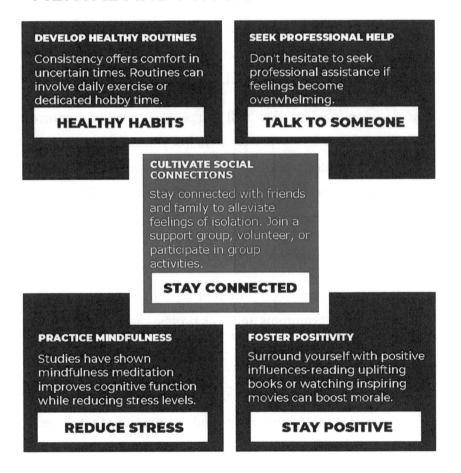

DEVELOP HEALTHY ROUTINES

Consistency offers comfort in uncertain times. Routines can involve daily exercise or dedicated hobby time.

HEALTHY HABITS

SEEK PROFESSIONAL HELP

Don't hesitate to seek professional assistance if feelings become overwhelming.

TALK TO SOMEONE

CULTIVATE SOCIAL CONNECTIONS

Stay connected with friends and family to alleviate feelings of isolation. Join a support group, volunteer, or participate in group activities.

STAY CONNECTED

PRACTICE MINDFULNESS

Studies have shown mindfulness meditation improves cognitive function while reducing stress levels.

REDUCE STRESS

FOSTER POSITIVITY

Surround yourself with positive influences-reading uplifting books or watching inspiring movies can boost morale.

STAY POSITIVE

Summing Up

When faced with seemingly hopeless situations like early-stage dementia, it can feel like everything is spiraling out of control. However, you must remember that you still have agency over your reactions. You can make life-affirming choices rather than letting the situation consume you.

It isn't wise to ignore early signs and hope that 'it'll get better'. Unfortunately, early-stage dementia progresses over time, so immediate intervention is essential.

Every decision made today will shape your reality tomorrow. Remember, knowledge is power; it helps you take better care of yourself and provides practical support during tough times. Equip yourself confidently to face whatever lies ahead with accurate information and a supportive community at your side.

Here is what your action plan might include moving forward.

- Educate yourself about different types of dementia to understand symptoms and seek professional advice if needed.
- Process your emotions and seek professional support while adjusting to this new reality.
- Connect with support groups and communities that share similar challenges.
- Adopt appropriate lifestyle changes to aid in slowing cognitive decline and disease progression.

- Establish a tailored daily routine to support independence and consider where technology tools can help.
- Openly plan for future scenarios; consider legal, financial and health care strategies and be prepared for changes to come.
- Seek professional help around issues like sleep disturbances or depression linked directly or indirectly to disease progression.

Living successfully with early-stage dementia requires patience – both from yourself towards others and, more importantly, towards yourself too! It will take time to adjust to changes happening within you mentally and physically; give yourself grace throughout this process.

Remember, don't hesitate to reach out to trained healthcare professionals at any time for additional help and support when you need it. Whatever it may be, for example: medication or health concerns, dealing with emotions, finding support groups, there are people there to help. You are not alone.

Key Takeaways

- *Dementia isn't only memory loss; it impacts every aspect, including emotional and physical well-being.*
- *You are more than just your diagnosis.*
- *Acceptance doesn't mean resignation*
- *There are many supporting resources – you are not alone.*
- *Emotional support from family members significantly enhances patient well-being.*
- *Patience becomes paramount when dealing with people diagnosed with this stage of illness.*
- *Home environment adjustments significantly reduce behavioral symptoms in early-stage dementia patients while enhancing their quality of life.*
- *Technology offers solutions that help to preserve dignity and make daily tasks easier.*
- *Regular social interaction is beneficial against cognitive decline in early-stage dementia.*
- *Despite cognitive decline, people with dementia can still perceive and experience feelings related to their dignity.*
- *Personal identity, autonomy, and relationships are critical factors in preserving dignity.*

4

Early Onset Dementia Challenges in Younger Adults

Sometimes life hits you in the head with a brick. Don't lose faith.

– Steve Jobs

A year into retirement, Carol noticed her husband, George, struggled with daily tasks. He was forgetting appointments and misplacing items more often than usual. The man who used to complete crosswords in record time now struggled to find words to express simple thoughts.

At first, they brushed it off as a natural part of aging. But when George forgot their wedding anniversary, a date he had never missed in 40 years of marriage, Carol knew something wasn't right. A visit to a neurologist confirmed their worst fears - George had early-stage dementia.

Early Onset Dementia Symptoms

Scientific research has shown that early-onset Alzheimer's, which affects people under 65, often presents differently than late-onset Alzheimer's. This difference is not just in age but also in symptoms and progression.

According to a study published in the Journal of Neurology, early-onset Alzheimer's often progresses more rapidly and can present with atypical symptoms such as behavior changes and difficulty with vision or language skills rather than memory loss. This can make diagnosing harder because these symptoms don't align with the traditional understanding of Alzheimer's disease.

Moreover, individuals affected by early-onset Alzheimer's are often still working or have young families, which adds another layer of complexity to their situation. The impact on their careers and family life can be devastating.

Therefore, if you or someone close to you is experiencing unexplained changes in behavior, language skills, or vision - especially if they're under 65 - it might be worth discussing these symptoms with a healthcare professional.

John's Story

John, a brilliant lawyer in his early 50s, was known for his razor-sharp mind and quick wit. He had always been the life of the party, a master storyteller who could hold an audience captive with his tales. But over time, things began to change.

He started forgetting essential court dates and misplacing case files. At parties, he would lose track of conversations or repeat stories he'd just told. John's wife noticed these changes and feared the worst, but John was only in his 50s - indeed, he was too young. Still, she insisted they see a doctor.

Their fears were confirmed when John was diagnosed with Early Onset Dementia (EOD). The news hit them like a punch in the gut; this wasn't part of their plan.

John's diagnosis is not as rare as you might think. According to Alzheimer's Association data from 2020, approximately 200,000 Americans under age 65 have EOD.

Unique Challenges of Early Onset Dementia

Financial Struggles: Living with EOD presents unique challenges compared to late-onset dementia. Many are still working when symptoms appear and may struggle financially due to lost income or medical costs.

Discrimination: John faced discrimination at work because people didn't understand that dementia isn't an "old person's disease". Colleagues grew impatient with him; clients questioned his competence. His career crumbled before him - a hard pill for someone who defined himself by his professional success.

Emotional Struggles: Friends drifted away because they didn't know how to interact with him anymore – all contributing towards feelings of isolation and depression common among those with EOD, according to studies such as one published in the International Psychogeriatrics Journal in 2016.

Despite these challenges, there is hope for people like John living with EOD. Research has shown that maintaining social connections can slow cognitive decline. This means it's vital for friends and family members to stick around and actively engage their loved ones suffering from EOD – playing games together or reminiscing about old times can make all the difference!

Moreover, don't hesitate to seek professional advice regarding financial planning or legal issues related to healthcare decisions - being proactive about these matters can alleviate some of the stress associated with this disease.

As for John? Well, despite everything, he kept fighting! With support from family and local support groups and cognitive therapy sessions, he managed to keep going daily– proving that while living with EOD is tough – it certainly isn't impossible!

Early onset dementia is a challenging journey for those diagnosed and their loved ones; however, staying active physically and socially while addressing practical concerns head-on will make navigating this journey less daunting.

Navigating Work-Related Issues

Pat Summitt, a legendary basketball coach for the University of Tennessee, was at the height of her career when she received devastating news. At just 59 years old, she was diagnosed with early-onset Alzheimer's disease.

Summitt had been a force on the court for nearly four decades. She held an impressive record: 1,098 wins and only 208 losses. Her reputation as one of the greatest coaches in history was indisputable. But suddenly, everything changed.

She first noticed memory issues and unusual behavior during games and practices. Her doctor confirmed what she'd feared - early-stage dementia. Yet, instead of stepping down from her head coach role, Summitt faced this challenge head-on.

Her decision to continue coaching wasn't taken lightly. Summit worked closely with her medical team to create a plan that allowed her to stay in her role while managing her symptoms. This included delegating more tasks to assistant coaches and using reminders and notes extensively.

Summit also decided to go public with her diagnosis, breaking down the stigma associated with dementia. In a statement released by the university, she said, *"I'm not going to let this keep me on the sidelines."*

Her courage inspired many others facing similar workplace challenges after being diagnosed with dementia or Alzheimer's disease.

Results of a study by the Johns Hopkins Bloomberg School of Public Health showed that adults who remain engaged in cognitively stimulating activities could delay cognitive decline onset related to Alzheimer's disease or other forms of dementia.

Continuing to work doesn't mean ignoring your diagnosis or pushing beyond your limits – it means finding new ways to do what you love while prioritizing your health needs.

Summit's story shows us that even after such a life-altering diagnosis, you can still contribute meaningfully at your workplace while maintaining your dignity and respect if given proper support and understanding by employers and colleagues.

Maintain a Sense of Normalcy

Maintaining a sense of normalcy and routine can significantly aid in navigating work-related issues after an early-stage diagnosis. According to a study published in the Journal of Occupational Rehabilitation, individuals who received an early-stage diagnosis and continued to engage in regular work activities reported better mental health outcomes than those who took extended leave. This is attributed to work providing structure, social interaction, and a sense of purpose - all factors contributing positively to mental well-being.

Communicate Openly with the Employer

The study also found that open communication with employers about one's condition was crucial for managing workload and expectations.

It allowed necessary adjustments or accommodations to be made, ensuring productivity without compromising health.

Therefore, if you've recently been diagnosed with a medical condition at an early stage, consider discussing your situation with your employer or HR department. It might seem daunting initially but remember - it's okay to ask for support when needed.

Try to Stay Engaged with Work

Additionally, try not to completely detach from your professional life as much as possible. Caring for your physical health and staying engaged mentally and socially through work are vital.

Practice Good Self-Care

Lastly, remember self-care outside of work hours. Regular exercise boosts mood by releasing endorphins - our body's natural feel-good chemicals. A balanced diet can also help maintain energy levels throughout the day.

Summing Up

Dementia doesn't discriminate based on age; neither should our understanding or empathy towards those affected.

If diagnosed with EOD, communicate openly with your workplace about your needs; stay engaged in work as much as possible; prioritize self-care outside of working hours; and remember that seeking professional psychological support is always beneficial when dealing with significant life changes like these.

Key Takeaways

- *Early onset dementia often manifests differently than older adults, making diagnosis difficult and delaying appropriate treatment.*

- *If diagnosed individuals are still working and have significant family responsibilities, they can experience additional stress and financial strain.*

- *Maintaining connections with friends and family members is vital. Actively engage in activities - playing games or reminiscing about old times can make all the difference!*

- *Seek professional advice regarding financial planning or legal issues related to healthcare.*

5

Lifestyle Changes to Slow Down Progression

 An ounce of prevention is worth a pound of cure.
— Benjamin Franklin

Living with early-stage dementia doesn't mean you have to accept an inevitable decline. Instead, by employing some key strategies, slowing the progression and enhancing your quality of life is possible.

The first step towards this is understanding that lifestyle choices are essential in managing dementia symptoms. This includes nutrition, exercise, medication management, cognitive stimulation activities, sleep hygiene, and stress management.

Dietary Recommendations for Brain Health

The food you eat profoundly impacts your overall health and well-being, including your brain function. When it comes to dementia, your diet can either be your strongest ally or your worst enemy. Certain foods are scientifically proven to boost brain health and slow down disease progression.

Think of your brain as a high-performance sports car. For it to run smoothly, it requires premium fuel – nutritious food. Research suggests that dietary patterns such as Mediterranean-style diets rich in fruits, vegetables, whole grains, lean proteins like fish, and monounsaturated fats from olive oil can help protect brain health. These are little superheroes fighting off harmful inflammation and oxidative stress.

Nourishing your body with wholesome foods supports overall health while helping maintain cognitive function.

A case study focusing on dietary interventions published in the Journal Of Alzheimer's Disease (Sofi, Macchi, Abbate, Gensini, & Casini, 2010) showed that individuals following Mediterranean diets rich in fruits, vegetables, and whole grains demonstrated slower rates of cognitive decline compared to those following other diet types – reinforcing our understanding about modifiable risk factors playing significant roles in managing this condition.

A diet including fruits, vegetables, lean proteins, and whole grains is crucial for maintaining good brain health. These foods contain essential nutrients like vitamins A, C, E, and K, Omega-3 fatty acids, and antioxidants that help prevent damage to brain cells. On the other hand, consuming excessive amounts of processed foods high in sugars and unhealthy fats can accelerate cognitive decline.

WHAT TO EAT FOR OPTIMAL BRAIN HEALTH

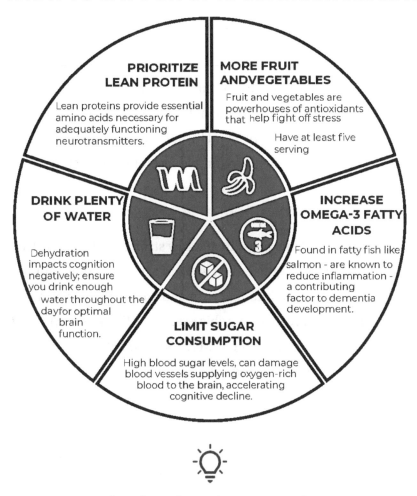

PRIORITIZE LEAN PROTEIN

Lean proteins provide essential amino acids necessary for adequately functioning neurotransmitters.

MORE FRUIT ANDVEGETABLES

Fruit and vegetables are powerhouses of antioxidants that help fight off stress

Have at least five serving

DRINK PLENTY OF WATER

Dehydration impacts cognition negatively; ensure you drink enough water throughout the day for optimal brain function.

INCREASE OMEGA-3 FATTY ACIDS

Found in fatty fish like salmon - are known to reduce inflammation - a contributing factor to dementia development.

LIMIT SUGAR CONSUMPTION

High blood sugar levels, can damage blood vessels supplying oxygen-rich blood to the brain, accelerating cognitive decline.

Tips for Changing Your Diet

- **Start small:** Make one change at a time until it becomes a habit, then move on to another.
- **Prepare ahead:** Meal prepping on weekends saves time during weekdays.
- **Enjoy what you eat:** Healthy food doesn't have to be boring!

> *"The food you eat can be either the safest and most powerful form of medicine or the slowest form of poison."*
>
> *- Ann Wigmore*

A healthy lifestyle doesn't stop at nutrition, though; regular physical activity is equally essential for maintaining good mental health, too! Physical activity pumps more blood through our bodies, including our brains, thus improving cognitive functions and mood stability.

Exercise Programs for Early-Stage Dementia

Just like watering plants helps them grow stronger, physical activity nourishes you brain. Regular exercise increases heart rate, pumping more oxygen-rich blood into the brain and enhancing performance. Tailored programs involving aerobic exercises (like walking), strength training (like lifting light weights), and balance activities (like yoga) are especially beneficial.

Benefits of Physical Activity

In the early stages of dementia, maintaining physical activity can be a game-changer. It's particularly beneficial for those dealing with cognitive challenges. The simple act of moving your body can enhance your memory, mood, and overall brain function.

Exercise is not just about keeping fit; it's also about engaging the mind and spirit. Incorporating regular physical activity into your routine stimulates your muscles and brain cells. This interaction between body and mind creates a powerful synergy that enhances cognitive function.

STARTING AN EXERCISE PROGRAM

START SLOWLY
Begin with light activites like walking or gardening gradually increase duration or intensity

MIX IT UP
include aerobic exercise, strength, flexibility and balance training , swimming , cycling , weights, yoga , tai chi

MINDFUL MOVEMENT
Dancing or martial arts are excellent choices requiring mental engagement and physical movement.

SAFETY FIRST
Consult healthcare professionals about starting an exercise program safely and recommendations on best exercises best suited for you.

CONSISTENCY OVER INTENSITY
It's more important to keep moving regularly than pushing yourself too hard during each session.

Research shows that people with dementia who engage in regular physical activity experience slower cognitive decline than those who don't exercise. (Tyndall, et al., 2018) They maintain their independence longer and enjoy a higher quality of life.

Moreover, exercise stimulates the production of brain chemicals that enhance the growth and connection of nerve cells. It also reduces risk factors such as high blood pressure which is a contributor to dementia progression.

But perhaps one of the most significant benefits of exercise is its impact on mood. Physical activity releases endorphins - 'feel-good' hormones - which combat depression and anxiety often associated with dementia.

If you find difficulty sticking to a routine or experiencing fatigue post-exercise sessions, consider working out in groups under supervision from trained professionals specialized in senior fitness programs.

Medication for Symptom Management

Medications don't eliminate the disease but can ease symptoms or slow progression. Acetylcholinesterase inhibitors or glutamate regulators are commonly prescribed by physicians based on individual needs.

Before starting new drugs, consult your healthcare provider about potential side effects or interactions.

Memory Techniques and Cognitive Stimulation Exercises

Cognitive stimulation activities such as puzzles or memory games help 'exercise' different parts of your brain, keeping them agile and healthy for longer.

The primary focus here is memory techniques and cognitive exercises designed to manage early-stage dementia symptoms and slow their progression.

The first principle to grasp is that your brain, much like a muscle, benefits from regular exercise. Cognitive exercises are designed to stimulate different brain parts, improving overall function and resilience. On the other hand, memory techniques help to retain and recall information more effectively.

Now let's delve into some cognitive exercises that can boost your mental agility:

Brain-Boosting Puzzles: Crossword puzzles, Sudoku, or jigsaw puzzles engage multiple areas of the brain simultaneously. They require concentration, problem-solving skills, and logic - all excellent workouts for your mind.

Memory Games: Simple games such as card matching or apps designed for memory enhancement can be beneficial, too. These activities promote visual recognition and recall abilities.

Creative Activities: Engaging in arts such as painting or crafting stimulates both hemispheres of your brain - enhancing creativity while sharpening fine motor skills.

Reading & Discussion: Reading books or articles followed by discussions with friends or family members can improve comprehension and verbal communication skills.

Cognitive stimulation activities like puzzles or learning a new skill may help delay memory loss by challenging your mind. Similarly, ensuring adequate sleep helps your body repair itself while reducing stress levels, known triggers for symptom flare-ups.

Improving Sleep Quality

Sleep is nature's most potent elixir, restoring us physically and mentally every night — research links poor sleep patterns with accelerated cognitive decline, suggesting good sleep hygiene is crucial for those battling dementia.

Scientific research suggests a strong correlation between the quality of sleep and the management of dementia symptoms. Studies have confirmed that disrupted sleep patterns can exacerbate cognitive decline in individuals who have dementia.

Tips for Better Sleep

- **Maintain Regular Sleeping Hours:** Your body follows an internal circadian rhythm that regulates your sleep/wake cycle. Going to sleep and waking at the same time reinforces your body's natural rhythm and promotes a better quality of sleep.

- **Create a Restful Environment:** Keep your bedroom dark, quiet and at a comfortable temperature. Ensure the mattress and pillows are comfortable and use earplugs or eyeshades if necessary. Avoid screens before bedtime.

- **Include Exercise in Your Daily Routine:** Regular aerobic exercise improves the duration and quality of sleep for older adults.

- **Limit Caffeine Intake:** Caffeine, especially close to bedtime can disrupt sleep patterns. Limiting intake during the day can contribute to a good night's sleep.

A study published in JAMA Neurology (Adam P. Spira, Alyssa A. Gamaldo, Yang An, & al, 2013) found that older adults with poor sleep habits had more beta-amyloid deposition in their brains - a hallmark of Alzheimer's disease. This implies that inadequate or disturbed sleep could potentially accelerate the progression of dementia.

Managing your sleeping habits is a key strategy in dealing with dementia symptoms more effectively. It's about getting enough hours and ensuring they are restful and rejuvenating for both body and mind.

Stress Management Techniques to Minimize Impact

Chronic stress acts like quicksand, pulling one deeper into cognitive impairment territory — managing stress through mindfulness techniques or controlled breathing exercises could positively affect mental well-being and slow symptom progression.

Mary, a retired schoolteacher, had always been an avid reader. She found joy in the worlds she discovered between the pages of her books. But as time passed, Mary noticed changes; she struggled to remember plot lines and characters. A doctor's visit confirmed what Mary had been dreading - early-stage dementia.

Refusing to let this diagnosis define her, Mary decided to engage in stress management techniques that could help slow down the cognitive decline associated with dementia and improve her quality of life.

Here are some practical ideas for managing stress to positively impact your journey with early-stage dementia and navigate this new reality.

MINDFULNESS EXERCISES

MINDFUL BREATHING

Reduce stress and calm emotions with slow deep breathing practice. Focus on the present, inhale deeply, exhale fully. Repeat for a few moments.

POSITIVE AFFIRMATIONS

Repeat positive affirmations to yourself, such as "I am strong and resilient."

MINDFULNESS MEDITATION

Take time to sit in stillness and focus on your breath or repeat a mantra

BODY SCAN

Focus your attention on different parts of your body and notice the sensations as you move through each one

Mindfulness: A Pathway to Calmness

A cognitive decline study completed by the University of California, Los Angeles (UCLA) (Wheeler, 2015) identified that individuals who regularly practiced mindfulness exercises showed less mental decline than those who did not. The researchers discovered that these exercises, including focused breathing and meditation, could potentially slow the progression of Alzheimer's disease.

Mindfulness practices help to reduce stress levels, which is crucial as high stress levels are linked to an increased risk of developing dementia. By lowering stress, you are effectively reducing your risk factors.

Therefore, incorporating regular mindfulness exercises into your daily routine could be beneficial if you're at risk or diagnosed with early-stage dementia. These practices don't need to be complex - simple deep-breathing exercises or meditative walks in nature can make a difference.

Start by setting aside five minutes daily for mindfulness exercises like breathing exercises or mindful walking. Gradually increase this time as you grow more comfortable with practice.

Spirituality too can provide peace and purpose for those diagnosed with early-stage dementia. A study published in the American Journal of Geriatric Psychiatry (Peter H. Van Ness Ph.D., 2002) revealed that patients who engaged in spiritual activities felt more connected to others and experienced less depression and anxiety.

Whether it's through prayer, reading religious texts, or connecting with a community sharing similar beliefs – all these contribute to maintaining mental health while dealing with such conditions.

Science shows us there's power in peacefulness – harnessing this power might give you the strength to face early-stage dementia.

Emotional Regulation: The Power of Positivity

It's natural for a diagnosis of early-stage dementia to trigger emotions such as fear, sadness, or anger. However, learning how to manage these emotions can significantly decrease your stress levels and enhance your overall well-being.

Positive affirmations are one way of achieving this emotional balance. These are short statements that you repeat to yourself throughout the day, which positively impact your mood and outlook.

Benefits of Art and Music Therapy

While there is no cure for dementia yet, therapies like these give hope where medicine fails - offering ways to reconnect with lost parts of oneself through creative expression while enhancing cognitive function at the same time.

When these creative therapies are integrated into daily routines (even if progress seems slow or demanding), they provide stimulation and moments of joy and connection. The sense of accomplishment achieved through artistic creation or musical engagement could never be matched by conventional treatments alone.

Therefore, these therapeutic approaches might be worth considering if you or a loved one is dealing with early-stage dementia. They enhance quality of life and contribute positively towards maintaining cognitive abilities longer.

A study by the Boston University School of Medicine (Hurst, n.d.) found that music therapy helps slow cognitive decline in patients with dementia. Listening to or singing songs, especially favorite and familiar ones, can provide emotional and behavioral benefits.

The science behind this is that musical appreciation and aptitude are among the last remaining abilities in dementia patients. Music triggers deep emotional recall; for individuals with Alzheimer's and dementia, music from their past can bring forth memories long since forgotten.

Music has also been found to reduce anxiety and depression symptoms.

Art therapy isn't just about creating pretty pictures or making clay pots; it's about using art as a form of communication and expression. According to a study published by The American Journal of Alzheimer's Disease (Chancellor, Duncan, & Chatterjee, 2014), art therapy enhances cognitive abilities and quality of life in Alzheimer's disease patients.

The study also showed that engaging with art can stimulate cognitive activity, foster self-expression, and reduce feelings of anxiety and depression. In this study, patients who participated in regular art therapy sessions exhibited improved memory recall, better concentration, and enhanced communication skills.

John and Sally – Moments of Joy Through Creativity

John was an older man, his hair white as the untouched snow on a winter morning and a bright twinkle in his eyes. Once upon a time, he had been an accomplished violinist. Now dementia, slowly but surely, started stealing away parts of him. John's daughter, Sarah, wasn't ready to let go just yet. She knew her father still had sparks of life left inside him, and she was determined to fan them into flames again.

Sarah remembered how much her father loved painting, set up an easel in John's room, and brought out all the paints they had at home. As John dipped his brush into vibrant hues of reds and blues, he began painting not just on canvas but also on the blank spaces dementia had created in his mind.

And then, one day, Sarah brought out her father's old violin. As John held the bow against the strings, familiar tunes started filling their home with memories of better times - each note acting as a beacon guiding him back towards himself.

Sarah realized that sometimes healing doesn't mean getting better; sometimes, it simply means remembering who you are despite what you've lost.

Sally was a woman of passion, her days filled with vibrant colors, laughter, and love. She had an infectious spirit that touched everyone around her. But then came the diagnosis of early-stage dementia. But Sally refused to let it define her.

She started painting again; each stroke on canvas was a testament to her resilience. Her paintings were abstract - bursts of color and emotion intertwined into one another.

Her son Jack took up the mantle to assist his mother in this fight against time and memory loss. He would sit with Sarah for hours at their old piano, playing familiar tunes from her past - songs she used to hum when he was a child.

Dementia might have taken away parts of John and Sally, but it couldn't steal everything. Even though we can't control certain things about our health or circumstances, we can still choose how we respond to them.

And for anyone out there battling similar struggles – know this: your worth isn't defined by your ability to recall past events or names or faces... it lies in how you live each day despite these challenges, how you find happiness in small things, how you continue making meaningful connections with those around you.

So here's to creating memorable moments every day – because while our minds may forget these experiences over time, our hearts will always remember how they made us feel.

Role of Occupational Therapy in Maintaining Quality of Life

Research has indicated that occupational therapy plays a significant role in maintaining functionality and improving the quality of life for individuals diagnosed with early-stage dementia.

A study published in the American Journal of Occupational Therapy (Piersol, Jensen, Lieberman, & Arbesman, 2018) found that people with early-stage dementia who participated in an individualized occupational therapy program demonstrated improved daily functioning, such as cooking, cleaning, and personal care, compared to those who did not. This increased independence significantly enhances self-worth and overall well-being.

Occupational therapists work closely with individuals to identify their unique needs and goals. They then develop personalized strategies to help maintain or regain skills necessary for daily living activities. These strategies may include memory aids, environmental modifications, or task simplification techniques.

Therefore, if you or a loved one is diagnosed with early-stage dementia, consider seeking the services of an occupational therapist. Their expertise can be invaluable in helping manage the condition effectively while preserving dignity and independence.

Dementia does not have to mean loss of autonomy or quality of life. Proper support from professionals like occupational therapists makes it possible to maintain high functionality and enjoyment.

Holistic Therapies and Early-Stage Dementia

Scientific studies suggest that holistic therapies, such as aromatherapy, can help manage symptoms of early-stage dementia.

When incorporated into a comprehensive care plan (alongside regular medical treatments), these holistic therapies can enhance the quality of life for individuals with dementia.

Keep in mind that every individual is unique, so what works best may vary from person to person. But don't underestimate the power of these simple yet effective therapies in managing this complex condition.

Reduce Anxiety with Pet Therapy

Scientific research has shown that pet therapy, particularly with dogs, can significantly benefit individuals with dementia.

According to a study published in the Journal of Alzheimer's Disease (Richardson, 2003), interaction with therapy dogs has increased social behavior and decreased agitation among people with dementia. The presence of these animals evoked memories and emotions, leading to improved moods and better communication skills.

The science behind this is fascinating. Interacting with pets increases levels of oxytocin - also known as the 'love hormone' - which helps promote feelings of trust, relaxation, and psychological stability. This can be especially beneficial for dementia patients who often experience anxiety and confusion.

So, if you or a loved one is struggling with dementia, consider introducing pet therapy. It could be a dog or other small pets like cats or rabbits. The important thing is that it's an animal you feel comfortable around.

Summing Up

Living with early-stage dementia involves taking care of physical health through regular activity and mental health by stimulating the mind while maintaining open communication about emotional well-being.

It means accepting change and adapting new strategies for managing everyday challenges. It's about investing time in activities that promote mental calmness, emotional stability, and physical wellness.

By understanding these needs and implementing the practical advice outlined in this chapter, you will ensure not just better management of symptoms but also an improved quality of life despite dealing with early-stage dementia.

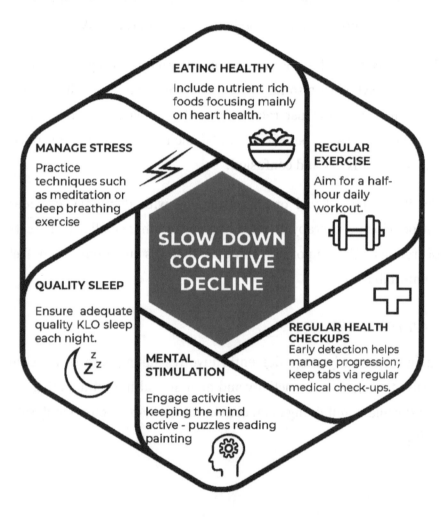

Everyone is different; what works for one person may not work for another. Consult a healthcare professional before making any changes to care plans.

While these techniques may seem simple enough to implement regularly into your daily routine, there may be days when motivation or frustration runs high; this is normal, given what you're dealing with right now!

On those tough days when progress seems elusive, remember:

- **Be patient with yourself:** Progress might be slower than expected, but don't lose heart.
- **Seek support:** Join a local support group for individuals dealing with similar issues.
- **Stay positive:** Practice gratitude and keep a journal to remind yourself of daily wins, no matter how small they seem.

And be patient, if you have trouble incorporating these changes into your routine, remember that small steps often lead to significant improvements over time.

When facing something extra challenging, such as severe anxiety or depression psychological support may be beneficial. Don't hesitate to seek professional help, especially when dealing with extreme emotional distress.

Key Takeaways

- *Lifestyle choices are indispensable in managing and slowing the progression of early-stage dementia.*
- *The food you consume directly affects your brain health; eating a balanced diet can slow down the progression of dementia.*
- *Excessive sugar intake accelerates progression towards dementia.*
- *Regular movement slows down cognitive decline.*
- *Engage in mindful movements that stimulate both body and mind.*
- *Be consistent – it's better to move a little every day than exhaust yourself once a week.*
- *Regularly engaging in diverse cognitive exercises and utilizing memory techniques can enhance brain health and slow down memory loss and dementia progression.*
- *Participate in creative tasks such as music, art, and gardening.*
- *Listening to favorite songs or singing with them can bring back precious memories.*
- *Medication is not curative but certain drugs can help manage symptoms.*
- *Adequate rest repairs bodily damage and effective stress control minimizes symptom flare-ups.*
- *Open communication is crucial – talking openly about emotions aids overall management.*
- *Remember, every step forward counts, no matter how small it may seem!*

6

Planning for Your Future Legal, Financial, and Health Considerations

> *In preparing for battle, I have always found that plans are useless, but planning is indispensable.*
>
> – Dwight D. Eisenhower

Preparing for the Future

Think of embarking on a long journey. You wouldn't just hop in your car without a map, snacks, and a good playlist for the ride. When dealing with early-stage dementia, it's the same principle. Even during this emotional whirlwind, planning is crucial for future legal, financial, and health considerations.

One critical aspect of this preparation is taking care of legal matters. For instance, creating or updating a will is essential to ensure your wishes are adhered to. Establishing a power of attorney provides peace of mind, knowing that someone you trust will decide on your behalf if you cannot. These legal documents may seem daunting, but they serve as a roadmap, guiding your loved ones when they need direction.

Financial planning is another vital part of this process. Costs related to medical care, insurance, and potential care facilities can add up quickly. By planning, you can ensure that resources are in place to cover these expenses. For instance, understanding your pension and insurance benefits can help you budget for future care needs. It's like packing the right snacks for your journey—you want to prepare so you won't go hungry.

Health considerations are equally important. This includes discussing care options such as home care, assisted living, or nursing homes. Each option has benefits and challenges, and personal preference is crucial in making this decision. It's akin to choosing the perfect playlist for your trip—you want something that suits your taste and makes the journey more comfortable.

Lastly, preparing for emergencies and having end-of-life conversations are critical yet often overlooked aspects of planning. Discussing these issues might feel uncomfortable, but doing so can alleviate stress and uncertainty. It's like having a spare tire in your car—it's something you hope you'll never need, but you'll be glad you have it if the situation arises.

Early-stage dementia isn't an easy journey. It is uncharted territory filled with twists and turns. But with careful planning and preparation—handling legal matters, managing finances, considering health options, preparing for emergencies, and having difficult conversations—you can navigate these waters more quickly and confidently. Think of this preparation as bracing yourself for the challenges; it's about enabling yourself to live fully despite them.

Planning isn't about giving up or succumbing prematurely to dementia; instead, it empowers you, providing control over how you navigate this journey called life.

Preparation today paves the way for peace tomorrow!

Legal Matters - Protecting Your Rights and Wishes

Firstly, let's tackle the legal maze. Imagine it as a labyrinth; each turn reveals new challenges and opportunities for protection and peace of mind. You may want to consider updating or creating your will, an essential document that puts pen to paper on your wishes concerning asset distribution after death. A living will or healthcare directive outlines your preferences regarding medical treatments if you cannot make decisions yourself, ensuring your wishes are understood and acted on.

It's also essential to consider appointing someone trustworthy as power of attorney. If you cannot do so yourself, this person will have the authority to decide on your behalf.

Likewise, an enduring power of attorney for finances allows someone you trust implicitly to manage your monetary matters if you become incapacitated. Lastly, guardianship supports those needing help with daily tasks such as paying bills or making medical decisions.

Taking legal precautions early can save unnecessary stress later.

Five Essential Legal Documents

- **Last Will & Testament:** A legal document expressing how your assets will be distributed after death.
- **Living Will:** Describes preferences for medical treatment if you cannot communicate or make decisions.
- **Enduring Power of Attorney (POA):** A trusted person appointed to handle your financial affairs if you cannot.
- **Health Care Proxy:** Like POA but specifically for healthcare decisions.
- **Guardianship Designation:** Specifies a person to make decisions for you when you cannot. Will be assigned by the if not specified by you in advance.

Steps for Legal Planning and Preparation

- Review, and if required, update your Last Will and Testament.
- Assign an Enduring Power of Attorney.
- Consider creating a Living Will.
- Discuss plans with your family and legal advisors.
- If in doubt about your level of cognitive impairment, get assessed by professionals before signing anything significant.
- Organize essential documents, bank statements, property deeds, insurance policies, etc., and keep them in one place for easy access.
- Informing any relevant authorities of your condition, such as DVM/DVLA, to continue.

According to Mary Radford, professor emerita at Georgia State University College of Law, "the importance of having these legal documents in place cannot be overstated." Without such preparations, "a court may need to get involved", which could be stressful and costly.

Legal Preparation and Planning: Q & A

Q. What are the initial legal steps after being diagnosed with early-stage dementia?

A. After a diagnosis of early-stage dementia, it's crucial to start planning and discussing these plans with your family and legal advisors. This includes reviewing and updating your Last Will and Testament, setting up a Power of Attorney, considering and preparing a Living Will or advanced healthcare directive.

Q. How can I ensure my financial affairs are in order if my condition worsens?

A. You can appoint a trusted person as your financial power of attorney who will manage your finances when you cannot do so. It's also wise to organize all essential documents, like bank statements, property deeds, insurance policies, etc., in one place for easy access.

Q. What is the role of an enduring power of attorney (EPOA) in managing my affairs?

A. An EPOA is someone you trust who is legally empowered to make decisions on your behalf when you can no longer do so due to mental incapacity. They can manage your finances, health care decisions, and personal welfare matters depending on what powers you grant them.

Q. How does a Living Will work, and how could it benefit me?

A. A living will or advance healthcare directive defines your wishes regarding medical treatment. It ensures that doctors follow your wishes about end-of-life care, which may include instructions about resuscitation efforts, use of ventilators, etc.

Q. What legal considerations should I think about concerning driving?

A. Laws vary by location, but generally, after a dementia diagnosis, there may be restrictions on driving, especially as the disease progresses, because it affects memory, reaction times, etc., making driving unsafe. It would be best to inform DMV/DVLA about the diagnosis; they may require periodic retesting.

Q. Can I still sign legal documents if I have been diagnosed with early-stage dementia?

A. Yes, people with early-stage dementia often still can sign legal documents like contracts or wills, but this depends on their level of cognitive impairment at that time, which professionals should assess before signing anything significant.

Q. How do guardianship laws work concerning those diagnosed with dementia?

A. Guardianship laws allow courts to appoint someone (a guardian) who makes decisions for another person (the ward) who cannot make informed decisions due to conditions like dementia.

Q. What happens if I don't prepare legal documentation before my condition worsens?

A. If no preparations are made beforehand, then once an individual becomes mentally incapable, they won't be able to decide things anymore and others would need court approval via the conservatorship/guardianship process, which can be lengthy and costly; hence, preparation is vital.

These steps indicate the significant actions to consider only. Everyone's circumstances are unique, and you should seek advice and assistance from appropriately qualified legal professionals.

Financial Arrangements: Preparing for Future Costs

Now imagine walking into an art gallery filled with abstract paintings representing your financial circumstances - pensions and insurance policies hanging side by side with future care costs and potential out-of-pocket expenses. Befuddling? Perhaps initially, but the picture becomes more apparent by focusing on one painting at a time - breaking down each element.

Insurance policies should be reviewed carefully; they are like well-tailored suits that need adjustments over time based on shifting needs. Pensions might seem like distant twinkles right now; however, clearly understanding them will illuminate what resources are available when needed most.

Financial planning is equally critical in this stage, as dementia care can be expensive due to its long-term nature. Be proactive in understanding potential costs such as home modifications, home-care services, or residential care facilities fees that could come up.

Early financial planning ensures resources are available when needed most

---

Consider discussing long-term care insurance options with a financial advisor experienced in eldercare issues. Scrutinize your existing health coverage and understand what services are covered under Medicare or Medicaid.

Steps in Planning Your Financial Future

- Review Insurance Policies and Pensions
- Investigate potential care costs.
- Consult with a financial advisor experienced in eldercare issues.
- Review existing health coverage to understand what is and isn't covered.

- Investigate public services provided and applicable eligibility criteria.
- Review retirement benefits
- Consider options for when savings run out.

These steps indicate the significant actions to consider only. Remember that everyone's circumstances are unique, and you should seek advice and assistance from appropriately qualified Financial Advisors and discuss options with family members.

Financial Preparation and Planning: Q & A

Q. What are the financial implications of an early-stage dementia diagnosis?

A. The financial implications can be significant and may include medical costs for ongoing treatment, care costs, potential loss of income, and possible need for long-term care insurance or other forms of financial protection.

Q. Can I still work after being diagnosed with early-stage dementia?

A. Many people with early-stage dementia continue to work for some time after their diagnosis. However, it depends on how quickly your symptoms progress and your job type.

Q. How does health insurance cover dementia-related expenses?

A. Health insurance coverage varies widely depending on the policy. Some policies may cover a portion of the cost of diagnostic tests, medications, and doctor's visits related to dementia. However, most health insurance does not cover home care or nursing home care.

Q. What are some ways to manage out-of-pocket healthcare costs associated with dementia?

A. Some strategies include exploring public benefits (for those who qualify), considering long-term care insurance, utilizing health savings accounts (HSAs) or flexible spending accounts (FSAs), and discussing payment plans or sliding scale fees with healthcare providers.

Q. How should I plan my retirement finances considering my diagnosis?

A. Consult a financial advisor who understands the complexities of planning for a future that includes a chronic illness like dementia.

Q. Are government programs available that can help offset some costs related to Dementia Care?

A. Yes! Some programs may cover certain long-term care services based on income levels and other eligibility requirements.

Q. **Are there any specific legal considerations that need attention post-diagnosis?**

A. It's crucial to update wills and ensure the power of attorney documents are in place while you can still make these decisions yourself.

Q. **How much does long-term care cost for someone with dementia?**

A. Costs vary greatly depending on location and level of care required but can range anywhere from tens of dollars an hour for home health aides and up to thousands of dollars per month for specialized memory-care facilities.

Q. **Is selling off property/assets due to impending high-cost treatments advisable?**

A. This decision should be made carefully in consultation with family members and financial advisors familiar with your situation.

Q. **What happens when personal savings run out – what options exist then?**

A. When personal savings run out, individuals may turn towards social security benefits they're eligible for, state-funded programs, non-profit organizations offering aid, family support, etc.

Care Options: Choosing What's Best for You

The question of care options is akin to Goldilocks' dilemma - searching for 'just right.' Some may prefer home care, which assists within their familiar surroundings. In contrast, others might find comfort in assisted living facilities that offer more support services without the full intensity of nursing homes.

Moving onto health care options, it's beneficial at this point to understand what levels of support might be required as dementia progresses - from home-care services in the early stages through assisted living facilities later when more intensive support might be needed.

However, just as seasons change, so too may our needs evolve, signalling it's time for a change in living arrangements. This could look like increased confusion causing safety concerns or physical changes, making daily tasks challenging.

But before we move on, let's discuss a common misconception about caring for a person with dementia.

> **"Only blood relatives can provide proper care."**
> This idea stems from outdated societal norms rather than factual information. Friends or other non-family members can be just as effective caregivers if they're willing and able!

> **"Professional services are unnecessary expenses."**
> On the contrary, professional intervention often leads to better-drafted care plans, ensuring a healthier physical and

emotional environment, thus making them worth every penny spent!

Try not to let such misconceptions cloud your judgments. Instead, investigate the facts about different options available in your community. Discuss these possibilities openly with family members who might be involved in helping coordinate your care later and work out what is best for you and your family.

Dr. Laura Gitlin from Johns Hopkins University suggests that "early conversations about potential future needs can reduce stress by providing clear plans that respect everyone's wishes".

Health Care Preparation and Planning: Q & A

Q. What care options are available for someone diagnosed with early-stage dementia?

A. Care options range from:

- *home care services* where a caregiver comes to your home to assist with everyday tasks.
- *adult day centers,* which provide social activities during the day.
- *residential facilities* like assisted living, which provide help with personal care and medications.
- *nursing homes* that offer 24-hour supervision and medical care.
- *continuing care retirement communities* that provide different service levels within one community.

Q. What are some advantages of home-based care for people diagnosed with early-stage dementia?

A. Home-based care allows individuals to stay in their own environment where they feel comfortable and secure. It can also be more cost-effective than residential facilities, depending on the level of assistance required.

Q. Are there any disadvantages associated with home-based care?

A. It could lead to isolation if not correctly managed since social interaction opportunities may decrease over time unless proactive measures are taken (like arranging visits). Also, depending on the progression rate of the disease condition, it might become increasingly difficult for family members/caregivers without professional training.

Q. When is it time to consider moving into a long-term care facility?

A. It's time when there are significant changes in behavior, such as:

- aggression towards self/others.
- inability to perform basic tasks like eating, bathing, etc.
- frequent falls/injuries due to confusion/disorientation.
- increasing medical needs beyond your or your caregiver's capability.

Q. How do I find a suitable long-term care facility (for my loved one)?

A. Start by identifying what specific needs you or your loved ones have, then research facilities that cater to those needs effectively. Visit potential places personally, check out staff responsiveness/facility cleanliness, etc., and consult healthcare providers/geriatricians who know about local resources.

Q. What kind of financial planning should we consider when exploring long-term care options?

A. You need to consider the costs involved, including ongoing monthly fees at residential facilities/home-care services charges, etc., check whether insurance policies cover these expenses partially/completely & explore Medicaid/Medicare benefits eligibility, too.

Emergency Plans: Be Prepared for The Unexpected

Many people believe that in the initial stages of dementia, there isn't much risk involved, hence no need for alarm or planning; however, , "Prevention is better than cure." By preparing now, you're setting up safeguards for future unpredictable circumstances associated with progressive diseases like dementia.

An emergency can arise at any time without warning; hence, it's prudent that you have an emergency response plan in place. This includes having available critical medical information (like allergies or current medications), identifying local hospitals equipped for emergencies related to dementia, and ensuring access within reach for emergency contact numbers.

An emergency plan for early-stage dementia patients can provide a safety net, ensuring the best care under the worst circumstances.

Why Do You Need an Emergency Plan?

In the early stages of the dementia, individuals an experience mild confusion or forgetfulness that can escalate into severe health or safety issues.

Consider this scenario: you wander off alone and get lost and confused. Without an emergency plan, this situation could quickly become a crisis. However, if adequately prepared, your family will know exactly what steps to take to ensure your safe return.

Creating Your Emergency Plan

Crafting an effective emergency plan can be likened to assembling pieces of a puzzle – each representing different aspects such as personal information, medical details, essential contacts, etc. Let's dive into each piece.

1. **Assemble Information**

   - **Personal Information** - should include full name, address, contact numbers, and any distinguishing features that might help identify them.
   - **Medical Details** - include medications taken daily, allergies, if any, and other relevant health conditions as well as dementia.
   - **Essential Contacts** - list all the necessary contacts, including phone numbers for family members', neighbors', and doctors'.
   - **Photograph** – carers and family members should keep recent photos handy, which could be extremely useful during search operations.
   - **Personal Preferences and Communication Strategies** –document some personal habits, preferences, and communication strategies that work effectively; it could come in handy for someone unfamiliar during emergencies.

2. **Utilize Technology**

   In our digital era, technology has extended its helping hand even towards dementia care management. GPS trackers can be attached discreetly to the clothes or shoes of individuals prone to wandering off due to confusion caused by their condition.

3. **When Things Get Tough**

   If things go south despite your best efforts, do not lose hope! Contact local authorities immediately, providing them with all necessary information from your meticulously crafted emergency plan while simultaneously reaching out to those on your essential contacts list.

4. **Share the Plan with Others**

   Here are some ideas of who to share the plan with or make aware that one exists.

   - Reach out to neighbors and local community services explaining the condition so they can assist if required.
   - Give a copy of the plan to everyone involved in the person's care.
   - Place copies in easily accessible places around the house.

The essence of crafting an exceptional emergency plan lies in its attention to detail and comprehensiveness. It's about being proactive rather than reactive when facing challenging situations brought on by dementia.

Giving thought today about potential problems tomorrow might save you from unnecessary stress while ensuring optimum care for your loved one battling dementia at its earliest phase.

End of Life Conversations: Facing the Future with Honesty

Finally, we come to what many may deem as the elephant in the room – end-of-life conversations (EOL). They're tough yet necessary discussions about treatment preferences during severe illness or life's end stage.

While considering end-of-life decisions earlier after diagnosis can be uncomfortable, doing so ensures that treatment preferences are respected when you may not have the capacity later.

John was a vibrant, healthy man of 65. He had recently retired from his job as a high school history teacher, looking forward to spending his golden years traveling with his wife, playing golf, and reading the books he never had time for before. But life has a way of throwing curveballs.

One day, while shopping with his wife Susan, John couldn't remember how to get home. It was an ordinary route they'd taken countless times before, but it was like navigating through unfamiliar territory this time. This incident began numerous forgotten moments that led them to consult a neurologist.

The diagnosis was early-stage dementia.

You could feel the chill in the room when they received the news. It felt like all their dreams for retirement were suddenly shattered into pieces. But despite this devastating revelation, there was something that kept them going - love and honesty.

They decided then and there that they would face this challenge head-on with open communication about what lay ahead - including treatment preferences during severe illness or at life's end stage.

Now you might be thinking – isn't it too soon? According to a study published in the Neurology Journal in 2018, patients diagnosed with early-stage dementia can still participate actively in decision-making regarding their future care and end-of-life wishes. The earlier these discussions happen, the better it is for everyone involved.

And so began their journey down this challenging road.

With courage and openness as their guiding lights, John and Susan started having these tough conversations about what kind of medical intervention John would want if he reached a point where he couldn't express himself anymore. They discussed do-not-resuscitate orders (DNR), feeding tubes, and hospitalization preferences – topics most couples avoid until it's too late.

They even consulted an attorney to put everything on paper, ensuring John's wishes were legally binding through advance directives like living wills or healthcare power of attorney documents.

These conversations weren't easy by any means; there were tears, fears surfaced, but each discussion brought them closer together than ever before.

There's no denying that dealing with such diagnoses is emotionally draining, but being prepared helps alleviate some stress associated with uncertainty about the future.

We often forget we have control over how we want our final chapters to unfold because we're afraid to confront our mortality head-on.

But embracing your mortality doesn't mean giving up hope—it simply means acknowledging reality so you can live fully in whatever time remains.

If you or someone close has been diagnosed with early-stage dementia or any other terminal illness—don't wait till it's too late. Have those heart-to-heart talks now when you can still make rational decisions without emotional duress clouding judgment.

Remember—end-of-life discussions are not just for patients nearing death—they are meant for all of us because we're all mortals navigating our way through life one day at a time!

End-of-Life Discussions: Q & A

Q. What critical points should be discussed when planning end-of-life care in early-stage dementia?

A. You may want to include the following points.
- preferred place of death,
- desired level of medical intervention (e.g., resuscitation, feeding tubes),
- pain management preferences,
- funeral arrangements,
- financial matters,
- legacy/heritage preservation.

Q. How can I initiate a conversation about end-of-life preferences with my family or my loved one diagnosed with early-stage dementia?

A. Start by expressing your love and concern, explain why it's important to discuss now while they can still express their wishes clearly, and reassure them that you want to honor their choices.

A. Seek support from therapists/counselors experienced in dealing with terminal illness/grief; join support groups where you can share experiences/challenges/solutions with others facing similar situations.

A. Consider preparing an Advance Healthcare Directive/Living Will, which outlines medical treatment preferences; Durable Power of Attorney for Health Care designates someone else to make health decisions if they become unable; Last Will/Testament details distribution of assets after death.

A. Discuss interventions like CPR/resuscitation, mechanical ventilation/intubation, and artificial nutrition/hydration - all may prolong life but potentially decrease quality.

A. Consider engaging palliative care specialists or hospice organizations; Alzheimer's Association offers resources/support; Elder law attorneys can guide you on legal/financial matters.

Q. **How can we ensure healthcare providers respect and follow my end-of-life wishes?**

A. Clearly communicate your loved one's wishes through advance directives/living wills; regular discussions with the healthcare team ensure everyone understands/agrees on goals/care plans.

Q. **Can you share some experiences on how families have handled this situation effectively?**

A. Experiences vary widely – some families find comfort in open discussion/planning ahead while others struggle due to cultural/personal beliefs around death/dying; professional guidance/support is often beneficial during the process.

Q. **When is the right time to start discussing end-of-life care after a diagnosis of early-stage dementia?**

A. The sooner, the better - ideally, when you are still capable enough mentally/emotionally to handle such serious topics/make an informed decision about future care/treatment options.

Q. How will the progression of dementia affect my ability to make decisions about my own care, and how can I account for this in our planning?

A. As dementia progresses, decision-making capacity declines. Hence, it is important to start conversations/planning early so that your desires are known/respected even when you can no longer articulate for yourself.

The Bottom Line: Taking Control of Your Future

When Marjorie was diagnosed with early-stage dementia at 62, she felt a whirlwind of emotions. Anxiety, fear, sadness - all these emotions swirled around her. Yet amidst this storm, Marjorie found a sense of resolve. Rather than being consumed by the dread of an uncertain future, she decided to take control and plan.

With the help of her family and a team of professionals, Marjorie started preparing for what may lie ahead. She organized her legal affairs, made necessary financial arrangements, and discussed potential care options. Her proactive approach gave her a sense of control over her life, easing the burden on her loved ones.

Being diagnosed with early-stage dementia undoubtedly presents many challenges, but taking proactive steps toward planning gives you control over how those challenges will be met.

By addressing key areas such as legal protections, financial provisions, and healthcare choices now – while still able –you can ensure that your rights are protected, resources maximized efficiently, and personal preferences honored throughout this journey, just like Marjorie did.

Key Takeaways

- *Legal documents should be updated immediately after diagnosis.*
- *Understanding potential costs related to dementia helps in better financial planning.*
- *Knowing different levels of support available aids decision-making regarding care options.*
- *Having honest conversations about end-of-life scenarios ensures personal wishes are respected even when communication becomes difficult later.*

7

Navigating Relationships and Emotional Support

 The greatest healing therapy is friendship and love.
                                    – Hubert H. Humphrey

Steering Through Emotional Waters

Think of a ship embarking on an uncharted journey. The crew is prepared, and the sails are raised, but the waters they sail into are unknown. This is how it can feel when you or a loved one is diagnosed with early-stage dementia. It's a journey into the unknown, where relationships become your compass and anchor.

Dementia doesn't just affect the individual diagnosed; it inevitably changes the dynamics within their circle of relationships. Firstly, there's the difficult task of sharing the news. This requires careful thought and sensitivity, as reactions can vary widely, from disbelief to empathy.

Secondly, a diagnosis of dementia often leads to feelings of isolation for the individual and their family. It's essential to actively fight against this by building a solid support network.

Thirdly, there's the delicate balance between maintaining independence and ensuring safety. As dementia progresses, simple tasks can become challenging. Adapting to these changes is crucial while safeguarding the individual's dignity and autonomy. For example, technology like reminder apps or GPS trackers can help maintain independence while ensuring safety.

Navigating relationships and emotional support when dealing with dementia is not always easy. Still, every journey is easier when you're not alone. Surrounding yourself with supportive relationships is like having a sturdy ship to keep you afloat. It won't make the waters less turbulent, but it will make the journey more bearable.

The Ripple Effect: Early-Stage Dementia and Family Dynamics

While dementia is often seen as the villain that robs a person of their memory, it's equally notorious for impacting family relationships. Imagine casting a pebble into a serene pond - the effect isn't limited to where the stone sinks; ripples spread out, touching every corner of the water body. Similarly, an early-stage dementia diagnosis doesn't just affect the individual; it reverberates through the entire family.

The initial shockwave that sweeps across everyone involved can be intense. Science shows that stress levels increase significantly in caregivers after such revelations.

There's no sugarcoating it - living with early-stage dementia will test your family bonds to their limits. Think of wandering into a maze without any maps or compasses, taking each twist and turn filled with uncertainty. But, you're not alone and help is always at hand.

Early-stage dementia does not only affect an individual but also creates ripples within familial relationships by increasing stress levels and testing bonds.

Early-stage dementia undoubtedly causes upheaval within families. However, navigating this challenging phase together could also result in stronger bonds forged amidst adversity, creating memories worthy of cherishing forever.

Tips for Navigating Family Dynamics

- **Open communication** - Gather around as a family and discuss what lies ahead openly and honestly. This may seem daunting, but it will clear the path to mutual understanding and collective decision-making later.
- **Adapting roles** - With time, roles within your family will need adjusting depending upon who has more bandwidth or resources to care for the person diagnosed with dementia.
- **Seeking professional help** - If things get overwhelming, see a professional therapist or counselor specializing in dealing with such situations.

Sharing Your Diagnosis

Living with early-stage dementia is a journey that requires courage, patience, and a strong support network. Sharing your diagnosis with others may feel overwhelming. You might fear the reactions of those around you or worry about becoming a burden. However, it's important to know that sharing your diagnosis allows the people that care about you to understand what you're going through and offer their support.

It's essential because once they know what's happening they can give you all the help you need.

"Dementia does not rob someone of their dignity. It's our reaction to them that does."

- Teepa Snow

Who Should You Tell, and How Much Should You Tell Them?

When deciding who to tell about your diagnosis, consider their relationship to you and how they can contribute positively to your journey. Some people may provide emotional support, while others might help manage practical matters such as healthcare appointments or financial affairs. Be honest but concise when explaining your situation; too many details might overwhelm them.

Tips for Sharing Your Diagnosis

- Share your diagnosis selectively based on potential positive contributions from everyone. Openness about your condition invites supportive actions from loved ones.
- Approach conversations about dementia respectfully, considering cultural differences. Respecting cultural nuances ensures everyone feels heard and respected as caregivers or supporters.
- Maintain open lines of communication regarding physical intimacy needs and concerns.

Cultural Considerations when Sharing Your Diagnosis

Cultural considerations are also crucial when navigating relationships post-diagnosis. Different cultures have varying attitudes towards dementia; some may view it as a natural part of aging, while others see it as an illness needing treatment. Understanding these perspectives helps in fostering mutual respect and empathy within diverse families.

In the Journal of Aging Studies (Jones, Chow, & Gatz, 2006), a study explored cultural differences in perceptions of Alzheimer's disease among Asian American families. The findings showed that language barriers often made it difficult for non-English speaking family members to understand the nature of the disease and its implications on daily life activities. A better understanding was fostered by offering translated materials or interpreters during discussions, leading to more effective patient care strategies.

Maintaining Your Sexual Relationship

Maintaining sexual relationships post-diagnosis is another delicate topic worth addressing. Dementia doesn't eliminate the need for intimacy and companionship, but communication becomes even more critical in maintaining healthy sexual relationships between partners affected by dementia.

If problems arise, like confusion or memory loss during intimate moments, reassure each other with gentle reminders or cues without causing embarrassment or discomfort.

Remember, despite how isolating early-stage dementia might feel sometimes, there are always hands reaching out, ready to offer comfort if only we let them know where we stand – that starts by sharing our story bravely yet thoughtfully with those around us who matter most!

Dealing with Feelings of Guilt

Scientific studies (Aldridge & Laidlaw, 2017) suggest that guilt and shame are common emotions when diagnosed with early-stage dementia. These feelings often stem from the perceived burden placed on family due to their increasing reliance on them.

These negative emotions can significantly impact the mental health of those living with dementia, exacerbating symptoms and potentially hastening cognitive decline. This emotional distress is detrimental to the individual and adds additional caregiver stress.

However, there's a silver lining here. Research has shown that open communication about these feelings between can alleviate some of this emotional burden. By expressing their fears and concerns, individuals with dementia may feel less isolated and more understood.

Furthermore, experts suggest that implementing coping strategies such as mindfulness exercises or therapeutic interventions like Cognitive Behavioral Therapy (CBT) can help manage these feelings of guilt and shame. These techniques shift focus away from negative self-perception towards acceptance and resilience.

So, when dealing with early-stage dementia, it's crucial to focus on physical health and emotional well- being. Don't hesitate to seek professional help if needed - therapists specializing in geriatric mental health can provide invaluable support during this challenging time.

It's okay to ask for help; doing so doesn't make you a burden but allows your loved ones to show their love through care. And always keep communicating – it's vital in maintaining solid relationships despite the challenges.

Building Your Support Network

> *"Never believe that a few caring people can't change the world. For indeed, that's all who ever have."*
>
> *- Margaret Mead*

A robust support network acts like a safety net during a high-wire act; you can bounce back even if you lose your balance momentarily.

Communication is paramount within any social circle; however, specific communication issues can arise due to cognitive decline linked with dementia, such as:

- Difficulty finding suitable words.
- Repeating questions/ statements
- Losing train of thought
- Misinterpreting conversations

These issues can lead to frustration or embarrassment among both parties involved. A compassionate support network fosters patience and understanding, allowing ample space for expression without judgment. In this haven, one isn't defined by illness.

Moreover, being part of support groups also provides access to resources (like therapist contacts), shared coping strategies (like memory aids), and offers invaluable emotional reassurance, boosting confidence levels while dealing with everyday tasks.

It is comforting to know that life continues beyond an early-stage dementia—with laughter amidst hurdles and warmth permeating chilly days—if you have allies beside you every step along the way.

Tips for Building Your Support Network

- **Identify Key Members**: Include relatives, friends, or neighbours willing to provide emotional and practical support.

- **Leverage Medical Professionals**: Regular interactions with doctors, nurses, and therapists offer expert guidance.

- **Join Dementia-Specific Groups**: Connect with those facing similar situations for understanding and empathy.

- **Seek Professional Caregivers**: In severe cases, professional caregivers can provide comprehensive assistance.

- **Be Patient**: Building relationships takes time, so allow bonds to form organically.

- **Utilize Technology Platforms**: Online forums and video conferencing enable connection from anywhere at any time.

Dealing with Feelings of Isolation

Jane was a lively woman, full of energy and zest for life. She loved gardening and could spend hours tending to her flowers or pruning her fruit trees. She was diagnosed with early-stage dementia a few years back.

One day, while sitting on the park bench under her favorite willow tree, she confessed to a friend, "You know," she began, looking at the children playing nearby, "sometimes I feel so alone."

These words hit Jane's friend hard. Here was this vibrant woman who had always been surrounded by friends and family, now feeling isolated because of her condition.

Jane explained how it felt as if there was an invisible wall between her and everyone else - one that seemed to grow thicker with each passing day. She would forget names or lose track of conversations, making social interactions challenging.

But then Jane did something unexpected; she started going out more often rather than less. She joined a local gardening club where people knew about her condition but didn't treat her differently.

She also volunteered at the community center, teaching kids how to plant seeds and care for them as they grew into beautiful flowers or tasty vegetables. This kept her active and helped forge new connections with people who saw beyond her illness.

Jane's approach to dealing with isolation wasn't easy nor immediate; it required courage and determination to step out from behind that invisible wall she felt confined within. Slowly and surely, Jane found herself again amongst old and new friends, engaging in meaningful activities that brought joy to her and those around her.

Isolation is not just physical distance from others but also emotional disconnection – feelings of being misunderstood or overlooked because of one's condition can further deepen this sense of loneliness.

In Jane's case, by actively seeking connection through shared interests or passions like gardening, you can bridge these gaps created by dementia – making sure you are seen for who you are beyond your condition.

It requires strength and courage to reach out when you feel most vulnerable. However, doing so can make all the difference in maintaining your sense of self-worth and belongingness amidst such trying times. Be assured that you are never alone unless you choose to be. Reach out and connect through shared interests or passions - reclaim your place among friends & family because YOU matter far beyond your diagnosis.

Your value lies not only in what you remember but also in what you bring forth –love, kindness, or simply a passion for nurturing life like Jane.

Balancing Independence with Safety

Mr. Thompson was a retired engineer and loved his independence. His wife had passed away years ago, and he took pride in managing his life independently. But after he was diagnosed with early-stage dementia and his symptoms started to manifest, things began to change.

He would often forget where he kept his car keys or even that he no longer drove. Sometimes, he'd wander off during our neighborhood walks only to be found hours later by a kind passerby from the next block over. Yet, through it all, Mr. Thompson insisted on maintaining his autonomy.

Mr. Thompson put a lot of effort into maintaining control over his life - there were sticky notes all around his house - reminders for everything, from taking medication to turning off the stove.

But one evening, he left the stove on after cooking dinner and dozed off in front of the TV. The smoke alarm alerted his neighbors, who rushed over just in time to prevent any major disaster.

It became clear that while Mr. Thompson's desire for independence was admirable, it wasn't entirely safe anymore.

This is where technology stepped in as a savior – simple devices like automated pill dispensers ensured medication adherence; GPS tracking systems provided real-time location updates ensuring safety during wandering episodes; smart home devices turned off appliances if left unattended for long periods - these innovations allowed Mr. Thompson to maintain some level of independence without compromising on safety.

However, implementing these changes didn't come easy – Mr. Thompson initially resisted, but with patient support in demonstrating how they worked and explaining their benefits, he gradually accepted their value and importance.

Introducing simple tools into daily routines and making minor adjustments around the home environment can ensure safety while retaining a degree of autonomy.

As we witnessed in Mr. Thompson's story, embracing change can be challenging. However, adapting our approach based on evolving needs leads to better outcomes for all parties – allowing family and carers peace of mind by ensuring safety while preserving dignity and a sense of self-worth for the person with dementia.

Balancing safety with independence when living with early-stage dementia requires adaptability, patience, communication, and sometimes technological aids. While it may seem challenging at first glance, gradual implementation of necessary changes coupled with understanding & respect towards an individual's need for autonomy can pave the way towards safe yet independent living conditions.

Coming to Terms with Grief & Loss

Grief is a profound emotion often associated with losing a loved one. But grief isn't exclusive to death; it can also surface in circumstances where there's the loss of health, independence, or cognitive abilities—as is the case with early-stage dementia.

When confronted with a diagnosis of dementia, you or your loved ones may experience an intense sense of grief. It's not just about mourning the future decline but also grieving for what's already been lost—the cognitive functions once taken for granted.

Scientific studies have shown that allowing yourself to grieve is crucial when coping with life-altering diagnoses. Bottling up emotions leads to mounting stress and poor mental health outcomes. Embrace your feelings—sadness, anger, frustration- valid responses on this journey.

Grief isn't linear—it ebbs and flows like waves on a shore, sometimes calm, other times fierce, but always moving forward.

In such moments, remember this quote by Rumi: "The wound is where the light enters you." The light here symbolizes acceptance—a critical part of dealing with dementia.

For people with dementia who find their distress escalating beyond normal levels—manifesting as severe depression or anxiety—it might be time to seek professional psychiatric help immediately.

It's necessary also that caregivers recognize their emotional responses towards changes brought about by dementia—a condition often referred to as 'anticipatory grief.' They, too, must take steps towards self-care, ensuring they stay resilient while providing support.

No two journeys through grief are identical; everyone experiences it differently at different paces—there's no right way, only your way!

Tips for Dealing with Grief

- **Acknowledge Your Feelings**: Acceptance begins by acknowledging your feelings without judgment. Imagine each emotion as a cloud passing over you—it arrives and then departs without causing harm unless we hold onto it too tightly.

- **Express Your Emotions**: Find outlets for expression—be it through talking things out or pursuing creative endeavors like art therapy, which has proven beneficial in managing negative emotions.

- **Seek Professional Support**: Reach out to professionals specializing in grief counseling if things get tough—they're equipped with tools designed to navigate these troubled waters safely.

- **Create a Support Network**: Having supportive friends and family around you who understand what you're going through makes this journey less lonely.

- **Practice Self-Care**: Exercise, good nutrition, and adequate sleep are essential for maintaining optimal mental health amid adversity.

Summing Up

A diagnosis of Early-Stage Dementia impacts the person with the diagnosis and significantly affects their family.

By understanding the whirlwind of emotions everyone is going through, communicating sensitively, and building a support network, the individual and their loved ones will be armed to overcome difficult times.

Key Takeaways

- *Sharing your diagnosis with loved ones opens channels for emotional support and understanding.*
- *Cultural sensitivity promotes harmonious relationships within diverse families living with dementia.*
- *Grieving after an early-stage dementia diagnosis is typical. Allow yourself space and permission to feel all emotions fully.*
- *Seek professional help if needed – don't ignore persistent feelings of depression or anxiety.*
- *Remember self-care—it's not selfish but essential in managing stress effectively while caring for someone else.*
- *Anticipatory grief experienced by caregivers needs acknowledgment, too—they require equal amounts of care, love, understanding, and patience from those around them.*

8

Navigating the Healthcare Maze

 Don't count the days; make the days count.
— Muhammad Ali

Think of standing at the entrance of a vast labyrinth. You know you must get to the other side, but the path is complex and filled with unexpected turns.

Your medical team is pivotal, much like a trusty guide would in our maze analogy. Choosing the right healthcare provider is paramount. For instance, a geriatrician specializing in the health care of older adults may be more adept at managing the unique challenges of dementia. They can provide a comprehensive care plan that includes managing medications effectively and coordinating with other specialists.

Drugs are like keys in our maze, opening doors to better health. But juggling multiple medications can be tricky. Taking numerous medications might increase the risk of drug interactions; therefore, understanding each drug's purpose, dosage, and potential side effects is crucial. It's like having a maze blueprint; you'll know what each key does and how it fits into your overall journey.

Let's remember oral health, an often-overlooked aspect. Poor oral care can lead to infection and exacerbate dementia symptoms or even heart disease. It's akin to a hidden pitfall in our maze that can be avoided with regular dental check-ups and good oral hygiene practices.

Living with early-stage dementia often means dealing with other chronic conditions, too. These might be different sections of our imagined maze, each demanding its own strategy and attention. Simplifying processes for taking medications and managing appointments becomes essential here, helping you traverse these sections without getting overwhelmed.

Choosing a Healthcare Provider

Choosing the right healthcare provider when you're living with early-stage dementia is a decision that carries significant weight. It's about finding someone who can prescribe medication or run tests and finding a partner who will help navigate this new terrain with empathy, understanding, and expertise.

It is different from picking apples at the supermarket. It's more akin to assembling an orchestral band, each member playing their part harmoniously but distinctively, making a sweet symphony out of a complex composition - your health.

When choosing a healthcare provider, it's essential to consider their experience and specialization in neurology or geriatrics, their approach towards patient care, availability for emergencies, location and accessibility of the clinic/hospital, and compatibility with your health insurance.

It is okay to take your time. Choosing your healthcare partners isn't a decision you need to rush. You should feel comfortable with your choice and confident in their abilities. Research different providers, ask for recommendations, and schedule consultations until you find the right one.

Your healthcare provider should be an ally. They should listen to your concerns without judgment, answer your questions clearly and patiently, and provide guidance based on your unique situation.

Choosing the right healthcare provider is more than credentials; it's about finding someone who listens, understands, and guides you through this journey.

Criteria for Choosing a Healthcare Provider

You can add your own criteria to the ones suggested here. Remember, the most important outcome is that you and your family are comfortable with the choice made.

Once you've chosen a healthcare provider you trust implicitly, remember that while they are experts in their field - no one knows your body like you do! Always communicate openly about any changes or concerns as soon as possible.

Enlisting a supportive family member to help with this process may be a good idea, especially if choosing becomes confusing or overwhelming.

CHOOSING A HEALTHCARE PROVIDER

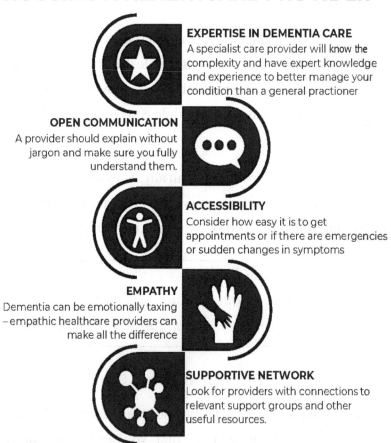

EXPERTISE IN DEMENTIA CARE
A specialist care provider will know the complexity and have expert knowledge and experience to better manage your condition than a general practioner

OPEN COMMUNICATION
A provider should explain without jargon and make sure you fully understand them.

ACCESSIBILITY
Consider how easy it is to get appointments or if there are emergencies or sudden changes in symptoms

EMPATHY
Dementia can be emotionally taxing – empathic healthcare providers can make all the difference

SUPPORTIVE NETWORK
Look for providers with connections to relevant support groups and other useful resources.

Understanding and Managing Medication

One key player in this ensemble is medication. Think of it as your first violinist setting the tone and pace for managing symptoms.

Medications can slow down the progression of symptoms in early-stage dementia by improving memory and cognition, managing mood swings or behavioral issues, and reducing anxiety or depression associated with dementia.

Understanding medications helps you know what to expect regarding benefits and potential risks. It allows you or your caregivers to recognize adverse reactions promptly if they occur and seek immediate medical attention.

Managing multiple medications can feel like juggling with fire while riding a unicycle on a tightrope – daunting yet crucially important. To make it less overwhelming, consider strategies such as using pill organizers marked with days/times, setting reminders on phones or alarm clocks for medication times, and keeping a medication log including dosage instructions and side effects noticed.

Managing Other Chronic Conditions Alongside Early-Stage Dementia

Imagine conducting your orchestra while other chronic conditions attempt their solos: diabetes strumming away on the guitar or hypertension beating loudly on drums. Managing these alongside early-stage dementia demands harmony through balanced care plans encompassing medication management, lifestyle modifications, and regular monitoring.

Regular check-ups are essential for monitoring all health conditions simultaneously. The healthcare provider may adjust treatment plans as needed, considering all health issues together rather than individually.

Regular Check-ups and Managing Appointments

In addition to these instruments tuning into your health melody, routine check-ups help monitor disease progression, much like music instructors guide students' growth over time, allowing them to hit high notes gracefully rather than stumbling blindly through compositions.

Routine check-ups allow doctors to monitor disease progression closely and make timely adjustments in treatment plans based on subtle changes that might not cause noticeable symptoms but could indicate disease advancement.

Tips for Managing Appointments

- Schedule appointments at the same time each day/week.
- Bring a family member/caregiver along.
- Have clear written instructions from doctors/nurses.
- Use apps that remind about appointments/medications.
- Organize transportation ahead of time.

Changes to Treatment Plans

But what if things go awry? If symptoms worsen considerably despite adhering religiously to treatment plans? Don't fret- there are encore performances in healthcare, too! A change in strategy may involve adding new therapies, such as cognitive stimulation therapy, or adjusting existing medications under professional guidance, ensuring the best possible outcomes.

As acclaimed neuroscientist Dr. Rudy Tanzi (Tanzi, 2005) once said, "Alzheimer's is not one disease...it's several diseases", alluding to its multifaceted nature requiring equally diverse approaches towards management - much like conducting an intricate symphony where every note matters!

Potential Health Problems with Dementia

People with dementia can often experience a few other common health issues. Understanding how certain conditions like incontinence and UTIs can affect your health will go a long way toward effectively managing overall well-being. These issues can exacerbate the symptoms of dementia and should be checked with doctors as soon as possible.

The Importance of Dental Care

Oral health might be overlooked, but it is vital in maintaining good health, especially in cases of early-stage dementia. Poor dental hygiene could lead to complications like gum disease, exacerbating dementia symptoms due to infection-induced inflammation.

Continence Problems

Incontinence is a common symptom among dementia patients, with up to 70% of people who have Alzheimer's disease experiencing some form of it. This can be due to various factors, including the brain's decreased ability to signal when the bladder is full, forgetting where the bathroom is, or being unable to get there in time.

According to a study published in the Journal of Alzheimer's Disease (Duffy, 1987), implementing a toileting assistance program can significantly reduce incontinence among dementia patients. The study found that by simply reminding and assisting patients to use the toilet every two hours during waking hours, incidents of incontinence were reduced by over 50%

When all your efforts are directed towards creating an environment that supports their needs (even if it requires extra patience and understanding), you provide them with dignity and comfort they might not otherwise have.

While dealing with dementia-related symptoms like incontinence can be challenging for you and your caregivers, evidence-based strategies such as scheduled toileting can make a significant difference. Always consult with healthcare professionals for personalized advice based on individual circumstances.

Urinary Tract Infections

Urinary tract infections (UTI) are a common occurrence in dementia patients as the disease progresses. This is due to several factors, including decreased mobility, increased use of catheters, and changes in the immune system associated with aging and dementia.

According to a study published in the Journal of American Geriatrics Society (Dufour, Michele, D'Agata, Daniel, & Susan, 2015), UTI can often exacerbate confusion and behavioral symptoms in individuals with dementia. Therefore, caregivers must be vigilant about preventing these infections.

One way to prevent UTI is by ensuring proper hydration. Dehydration can lead to concentrated urine, which creates an environment conducive to bacteria growth. A study from the University of Texas Southwestern Medical Center found that increasing fluid intake reduces the risk of UTI.

Maintaining good personal hygiene, especially around the genital area, is vital as it prevents bacteria from entering the urinary tract. Caregivers should also be aware of any changes in behavior or increased confusion, as this could indicate a possible infection.

Regular medical check-ups are essential, too, as they allow early detection and treatment of UTI before they worsen cognitive symptoms.

Summing Up

Assembling a great, supportive, and collaborative team of medical experts, having regular check-ups, and understanding your medications, side effects, and interactions are all essential to ensure the best care in monitoring and managing your health and disease progression effectively. This should include making sure that doctors develop a tailored care plan that incorporates your specific needs not only for early-stage dementia but also for any other existing chronic medical problems. Setting up simple processes using practical tools to make taking medication easy and ensuring that you remember and are prepared for medical appointments takes the stress out of juggling all the elements involved.

With the help of your caregivers, if needed, learn about your treatment and work with your medical team. Maintain open and honest communications; never ignore any new symptoms, whether related to early-stage dementia or not; continuously checking with your doctors is essential to manage your well-being in the best possible way.

Key Takeaways

- *Look for specialized knowledge in dementia care when considering potential providers.*
- *Balance care plans when managing other chronic conditions alongside early-stage dementia.*
- *Regular check-ups are essential for tracking disease progression.*
- *Be ready for strategy adjustments should symptoms worsen significantly despite current treatment plan adherence.*
- *Understand potential side effects of medications.*
- *Simplify medication management using various tools.*
- *Genuine empathy from caregivers is integral in managing emotional stress related to disease progression.*
- *A solid supportive network, including support groups, can prove invaluable as circumstances change due to disease progression.*

9

The Essential
Caregiver's Guide

" *Taking good care of YOU means the people in your life
will receive the best of you rather than what's left of you.*
— Karl Lagerfeld

Dementia is not just a disease; it's a profound shift in reality for both
patient and caregivers. The progressive cognitive decline and changes
in behavior affect not only the person diagnosed but also those around
them, especially family members who often become caregivers.

In the early stages of dementia after a diagnosis, life can seem like
uncharted territory. As a caregiver, you might feel you are wandering
alone in a labyrinth with no exit in sight. It is essential to focus on
your loved one and also treat yourself with kindness, compassion,
understanding, and forgiveness as you navigate loving and caring for
someone diagnosed with dementia.

Caregiving without self-care can lead to burnout. Caregivers often overlook their own needs while caring for someone else. You may find yourself feeling overwhelmed with caring for someone with dementia while also juggling work and family commitments and experiencing stress-related health problems. Remember that if you burn out, it not only does not serve you at all but leaves you unable to give the best to your family, work, and the person with dementia. Looking after yourself is NOT selfish; it is essential and the best thing you can do for yourself and everyone else.

As much attention must be paid to the caregiver's well-being as is given to the patient.

Prioritizing Self-Care: Essential, not Selfish

Research shows that caregivers are at increased risk of high blood pressure, heart disease, and a weakened immune system. These issues can severely impact their ability to provide care effectively when neglected. (Schulz & Sherwood, 2008) (Shaw, et al., 1999)

For example, in Mrs. Johnson's story, she was caring for her husband, who had early-stage dementia, while juggling her job as an elementary school teacher. She ignored her own health until she had a stroke due to unchecked hypertension caused by overwhelming stress levels.

Self-care isn't selfish; instead, it ensures that you're fit enough physically and mentally to take on what could be one of your life's most challenging roles – providing compassionate care for someone living with dementia.

According to statistics from the Alzheimer's Association Report 2019:

- Nearly half (48%) of care contributors have felt stressed in the previous five years.
- One-third (33%) say their health has worsened over time owing to caregiving responsibilities.

These statistics indicate the risks caregivers face and highlight their need to look after themselves and get help when needed.

Analyzing Mrs. Johnson's case further reveals how important it is for caregivers to focus on their loved one's needs and theirs. Ignoring personal needs leads down a path where both parties suffer adversely.

Remember that your loved one is probably struggling with guilt about being a burden on you, and seeing you stressed, exhausted, and burning out will only add to this, causing stress and anxiety, and increasing risk factors for further decline. One of the best things you can do for them is look after yourself.

What Does Caregiver Self-Care Look Like?

Studies suggest that taking time out for self-care activities can significantly reduce stress levels among caregivers, leading them toward better mental health outcomes.

Self-care activities can include:

- regular physical exercise - a healthy body leads to more beneficial emotions.
- engaging in hobbies or interests outside caregiving
- maintaining social connections

- taking frequent breaks from caregiving responsibilities - short breaks throughout the day and longer respite breaks when needed. Seek respite care if needed.
- maintaining a healthy diet
- getting enough sleep
- practicing mindfulness or meditation techniques to manage stress
- seeking support from friends or professional counselors

Now, I hear your frustrated scream, "I'm already overwhelmed! How do I fit more in?"

But remember, you cannot pour from an empty cup. Take care of yourself first so you can effectively take care of others.

When you focus all your actions on caring for another person, it's essential to remember that your health matters, too. You can provide better care if you're physically fit and mentally strong.

How Caregivers Can Make Time for Self-Care

There is no doubt of the value of self-care for caregivers, but how on earth do you find the time?

Studies show that regular self-care activities lower levels of stress and burnout and can prevent depression or anxiety disorders. Furthermore, participating in these activities means caregivers are more effective because they have more energy and patience to devote to their loved ones.

So, prioritize some 'me' time every day - even if it's just 15 minutes spent reading a book or walking around the block. This is not selfish; it's necessary for you and those depending on your care.

If you're sometimes struggling due to emotional exhaustion or lack of personal time, use respite services or ask family members or friends for help.

Professional therapists specializing in caregiver stress management can equip you with strategies to deal effectively with daily challenges while tending to someone's dementia.

Self-Care Action Plan

- **Step #1:** Start acknowledging caregiving's emotional and physical toll on you – denial will only exacerbate the situation.
- **Step #2:** Prioritize your self-care.
- **Step #3:** Take breaks, schedule 'me-time', engage in hobbies/interests keep your mind engaged and relaxed.
- **Step #4:** Don't hesitate to seek help – reach out to friends/family professional organizations that offer support services specifically for caregivers' individuals affected by dementia.

Remember, ignoring your well-being while caring for your loved one with Early-Stage Dementia is a disservice to yourself and your loved one, who is counting on you to stay strong and resilient.

The Balancing Act: Time for Yourself and for Others

It was a brisk winter morning, and Mary was sitting in the corner of a bustling café, her eyes fixed on the steaming cup of coffee that sat untouched before her. Her husband, John, had recently been diagnosed with early-stage dementia, and she was now his primary caregiver.

Mary was exhausted. Not just physically tired from the sleepless nights but emotionally drained from seeing the man she loved slowly lose himself to this cruel disease. Despite this, she remained determined to provide John with the best care possible.

Mary and John had a daily routine; they would start each day with a walk around their neighborhood park and breakfast at their favorite diner. In the afternoon, they would engage in memory-stimulating activities like puzzles or reading old letters together. Mary's entire world revolved around John's needs and well-being.

When asked about what she did for herself during these days filled with caregiving duties, she looked puzzled, as if self-care was alien to her. Countless caregivers like Mary are so engrossed in providing for their loved ones that they neglect their needs. They are so focused on keeping up with doctor's appointments and medication schedules that they lose sight of other essential aspects of life – personal hobbies, social interactions, and, most importantly, self-care.

It is vital to balance caring for your loved one and caring for yourself. It's easy to overlook the signs of burnout, such as constant fatigue or feeling overwhelmed, until you are already completely worn out.

Mary started gradually incorporating some self-care strategies into her routine - taking small breaks throughout the day while John rested or involving their children more actively in his care plan, which allowed her some free time.

Over time, these tiny changes significantly changed Mary's physical health. They improved her emotional well-being, making her more effective as John's caregiver.

The journey through dementia is undeniably challenging for those diagnosed and those who love them dearly enough to become caregivers; however, remembering to prioritize self-care amidst all the other responsibilities will benefit both of you in the long run.

Managing Emotions in Caregiving

Scientific studies suggest that anger or resentment towards someone you care for with early-stage dementia is common and perfectly normal.

Research published in the Journal of Applied Gerontology (Wylie, 2014) found that caregivers often experience negative emotions, including frustration, guilt, and resentment. These emotions come up mainly due to the challenging nature of caregiving tasks and the emotional strain of watching a loved one's cognitive abilities decline.

Thes feelings care harmful for your mental health. The study found that caregivers who reported higher levels of anger were more likely to experience symptoms of depression and anxiety. However, allowing these emotions to take control can lead to burnout and impact the quality of your care.

Acknowledging these feelings with compassion for your situation rather than suppressing them is a critical first step as well as an act of self-care. Accepting that your emotions are a valid, normal and temporary responses to a challenging situation allows you to manage them more effectively.

The Vicious Cycle of Resentment, Guilt, and Shame

The Cycle of Resentment-Guilt-Shame (CRGS) is an insidious loop in which many caregivers find themselves trapped. You may resent your situation or even the person you care for, leading to guilt about harboring such feelings. This guilt then transforms into shame - a deep-seated belief that you're somehow failing in your role as a caregiver.

Breaking free from this cycle requires self-compassion and forgiveness - what we'll call the "Compassionate Break." Acknowledge that your feelings are valid and understand they don't make you a lousy caregiver or person. Forgive yourself for any perceived shortcomings or mistakes; they're part of being human.

Tips for Cultivating the Compassionate Break

- **Identify Emotions:** Recognize your feelings without judgment, accepting them as natural responses to stress.
- **Practice Self-Compassion:** Show yourself the same kindness you'd offer a friend in similar circumstances.
- **Forgive Yourself:** Understand that mistakes are human, and forgiving yourself is essential.
- **Set Boundaries:** Learn to say no when needed and prioritize your self-care needs to reduce this frustration.
- **Seek Support:** Reach out to friends, family, or professionals for assistance. Consider caregiver support groups or online forums for shared experiences and coping strategies.
- **Practice Mindfulness Techniques:** Stay present-focused to reduce stress and avoid dwelling on past regrets or future worries. Even a simple 3-minute breathing exercise can help you find calm and regain perspective.

Finally, remember this. You are allowed to feel angry or resentful sometimes - what matters most is how you handle these emotions. Reach out for support when needed, prioritize self-care, and remember that by taking care of yourself first, you'll be better equipped to care of the people you love.

Finding Respite Care Services

Your role as a caregiver is critical in supporting your loved one. However, it's equally important to remember that you also need care and support; this is where respite care services come into play. Respite care offers temporary relief for primary caregivers, providing short-term care services that help to reduce stress, restore energy, and promote balance.

Take Martha, for example. Martha was a woman of immense strength and resilience. At 65, she was the primary caregiver for her husband, John, who had been diagnosed with early-stage dementia. Martha's days were filled with tasks to keep John comfortable and safe while managing her health concerns.

The love between Martha and John was palpable; they had weathered storms together for over 40 years. But this new challenge seemed too much, even to Martha's indomitable spirit. She felt alone in her struggle as friends didn't quite understand what it meant to be a caregiver for someone with dementia.

"Caregiving is not just about taking care of physical needs," said Dr Laura Gitlin from Johns Hopkins University during an interview on NPR (Gitlin D. L., 2015). *"It also involves emotional support, decision making, coordinating care, and managing difficult behaviors."*

One day, while attending a local community meeting, she heard about respite care services – short-term relief options designed specifically for people like her - caregivers who need a break without compromising their loved one's well-being.

Respite care could take various forms: adult daycare centers where trained professionals would engage John in stimulating activities or temporary homecare assistance that allowed Martha some time off from caregiving duties.

Excited by this discovery, Martha explored options available within her locality and found several suitable facilities offering programs tailored towards individuals with dementia.

With the help of these services, she managed to carve out regular periods of rest for herself - whether it was catching up on sleep or simply enjoying some quiet moments at the park nearby.

She shared her experiences at subsequent community meetings, passionately advocating respite care services to other caregivers like herself.

Seeking help is not a weakness; it does not imply failing at caregiving duties; nor does it mean surrendering control; instead, it shows strength in recognizing when you need support and taking action to find it.

"You are allowed to be both a masterpiece and work-in-progress simultaneously."

- Sophia Bush

Steps to Finding Respite Care

Use these steps to find the right respite care services for your needs. If it takes time take some time - don't panic! Ask questions when unsure about something, seek professional advice, or join support groups to learn from other caregivers' experiences.

STEPS TO FINDING RESPITE CARE

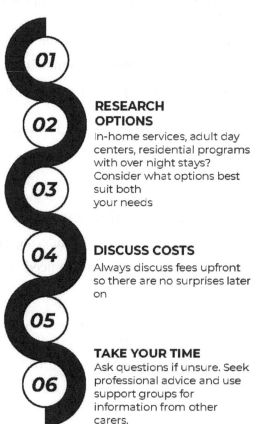

IDENTIFY YOUR NEEDS

Identify exactly what you need help with. Assistance with daily tasks like bathing and dressing or administering medication?

01

02

RESEARCH OPTIONS

In-home services, adult day centers, residential programs with over night stays? Consider what options best suit both your needs

EVALUATE PROVIDERS

Check qualifications, reputation and client reviews of potential providers. Visit facilities and check references.

03

04

DISCUSS COSTS

Always discuss fees upfront so there are no surprises later on

TRIAL RUN

Do a trial run to ensure the right fit before committing to a particular provider or service type.

05

06

TAKE YOUR TIME

Ask questions if unsure. Seek professional advice and use support groups for information from other carers.

Dealing with Challenging Behavior

"Remember: The person who has Alzheimer's disease did not ask for it – he or she would have chosen another path if possible."

- Paula Spencer Scott

As a caregiver, dealing with challenging behavior in loved ones with dementia can be difficult. The unpredictability of the disease often leaves you feeling overwhelmed and emotionally drained. However, understanding that these behaviors are not intentional but disease symptoms, can help you approach them with patience and compassion.

Dementia alters one's perception of reality, leading to confusion and frustration, often expressed through aggressive or disruptive behavior. Your loved one may become uncooperative, paranoid, or even physically violent. These behaviors are not deliberate but merely their way of communicating discomfort or distress.

To manage such situations effectively, try to identify triggers for these behaviors - it could be an unfamiliar environment is confusing or perhaps physical discomfort like hunger or fatigue. Once you've identified potential triggers, work towards eliminating them or finding ways to distract your loved one when they occur.

Understanding the cause of the behavioral changes is critical to managing them effectively.

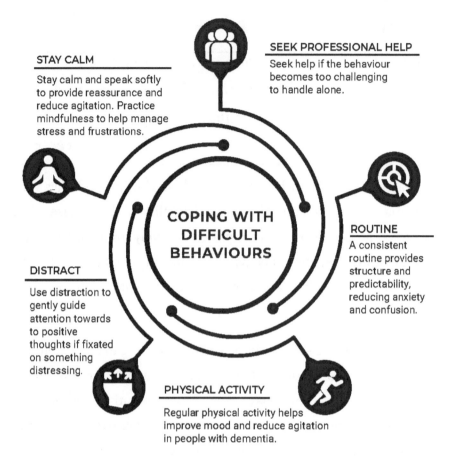

STAY CALM

Stay calm and speak softly to provide reassurance and reduce agitation. Practice mindfulness to help manage stress and frustrations.

SEEK PROFESSIONAL HELP

Seek help if the behaviour becomes too challenging to handle alone.

COPING WITH DIFFICULT BEHAVIOURS

ROUTINE

A consistent routine provides structure and predictability, reducing anxiety and confusion.

DISTRACT

Use distraction to gently guide attention towards to positive thoughts if fixated on something distressing.

PHYSICAL ACTIVITY

Regular physical activity helps improve mood and reduce agitation in people with dementia.

If, despite employing all these strategies, you still find yourself struggling with your loved one's behavior, there are additional steps you might consider:

- Join support groups where other caregivers share their experiences.
- Attend workshops about caring for individuals with dementia.
- Consider respite care services to take a well-deserved break.

Joining a Support Group

Scientific studies suggest that joining a support group has significant emotional and physical benefits for caregivers.

Research (Mittelman, Roth, Coon, & Haley, 2004) (Dieh, Mayer, Förstl, & Kurz, 2003) has found that caregivers who participate in support groups experience less stress and depression than those who do not. The shared experiences and advice from others can alleviate feelings of isolation and provide practical tips for managing care.

Furthermore, research has shown that participating in such groups can lead to better health outcomes for the caregiver. A study by the University of California found that caregivers who attended support groups had lower levels of inflammation markers in their blood, suggesting less risk of chronic diseases like heart disease and diabetes.

So, compelling evidence supports the idea that joining a caregiver support group could be beneficial.

When caring for someone with early-stage dementia, it's easy to feel overwhelmed and alone. By connecting with others who understand your struggles, you can gain emotional relief and valuable insights. Even if it initially feels difficult or uncomfortable, attending these meetings could significantly improve your well-being and ability to provide care.

In conclusion, don't underestimate the power of shared experiences. Contact local hospitals or community centers to find a caregiver support group near you. It may just be one of the best decisions you make for yourself -and your loved one.

Communicating Effectively

Science has shown that effective communication with people with dementia can significantly improve their quality of life and reduce feelings of isolation.

Studies (Collins, Anna Hunt, Martyr, Pentecost, & Clare, 2022) have found that personalized and empathetic communication alleviates symptoms of depression and anxiety in dementia patients. The research suggests that when caregivers use clear, simple sentences, maintain eye contact, and express empathy toward the person's experiences, it can profoundly impact their emotional well-being.

Furthermore, the Alzheimer's Association (Communication and Alzheimer's, n.d.) recommends maintaining eye contact during conversations as it helps to keep the person focused on the exchange. They also suggest avoiding distractions such as TV or radio noise, which could confuse or distract them.

Therefore, it is crucial to be patient and understanding when communicating with someone with dementia.

Instead of correcting them whenever they forget something or get confused - which can cause distress - try redirecting the conversation positively. For instance, if they struggle to remember a recent event, you could gently steer the conversation toward happier memories from their past.

Moreover, non-verbal cues such as body language and tone of voice play an important role too. A warm smile or gentle touch can provide reassurance even when words fail.

So, while dealing with dementia is undoubtedly challenging for both parties involved, adopting these scientifically-backed communication strategies will make interactions less stressful and enhance the bond between you.

Remember that the person behind the disease still needs your love and understanding more than ever. Your compassion and practical communication skills can make a difference in their lives.

These strategies may improve communication and enhance their quality of life by reducing frustration and confusion often associated with dementia.

"People with Alzheimer's do not move 'into' another world; they simply see this one differently."

- Naomi Feil

Quick Tip: Try to see the world from their perspective instead of trying to bring them back into yours.

Tips for Communication

- Keep your language simple.
- Maintain eye contact.
- Minimize background noise.
- Use non-verbal cues like gestures or visual aids.

Advocacy and Rights

> *"Dementia doesn't rob someone of their dignity; it's our reaction to them that does."*
>
> *- Teepa Snow*

Scientific research has shown that people with early-stage dementia can significantly benefit from being actively involved in decisions about their care and life.

A study published in Journal of Aging Studies (Fetherstonhaugh, Tarziaa, & Nay, 2012) found that people with early-stage dementia who were allowed to participate in decision-making reported higher quality of life, improved mental health, and a greater sense of dignity. They felt more valued and less isolated, which is crucial for managing this challenging condition.

On the other hand, those not included in these processes often experienced feelings of frustration, worthlessness, and depression. These findings suggest that maintaining a level of autonomy can play a significant role in enhancing well-being among individuals with early-stage dementia.

Therefore, it's important to advocate for the rights of people with early-stage dementia to be involved in decisions about their lives as much as possible. It's not just about ethical considerations; there are tangible benefits for their mental health.

Inclusion should extend beyond healthcare decisions to encompass all aspects of daily living – such as choosing what to wear or eat – no matter how trivial they seem. Doing so reinforces their self-worth and contributes to their overall well-being.

Just because someone has been diagnosed with dementia doesn't mean they've lost all ability to choose or express preferences. As an advocate or caregiver, your role is crucial in maintaining their voice throughout this time.

Summing Up

Let's be honest; caring for someone with a disease like dementia is challenging. It is not only the stress of worrying about the person you love and what will happen to them in the future, it is coping with the family dynamics around their condition, making sure they are safe, looked after, and supported, all while carrying on with your own work and family life as best you can.

It can be physically, mentally, and emotionally exhausting and draining.

First and foremost, remember that *taking care of yourself isn't selfish*; instead, it equips you better mentally and physically to provide optimal care for of the person with dementia and others in your life.

You are only human, and no matter how much you love the person you are caring for, there will be times when it feels too much. You will feel overwhelmed, angry, resentful, bitter, stressed, at the end of your rope; take your pick! Instead of beating yourself up – imagine you are listening to a friend; what would you say to them? Find empathy, compassion, and forgiveness for yourself, and give yourself a pat on the back for what you do and give to others daily. You are doing your best, and no one can expect more – not even you.

And please don't wait until you are burning out to follow the advice in this chapter. Set some boundaries, prioritize yourself; make self-care a part of your routine, and go on providing great care for the people who depend on you.

Key Takeaways

- *Self-care is not selfish; it is crucial as a caregiver.*
- *Caregivers feeling strong negative emotions is normal. Self-compassion and forgiveness are vital tools in breaking free from negative emotional cycles.*
- *Stay healthy - regular physical activity and a healthy diet contribute towards emotional well-being.*
- *Seeking support through therapy, friends, family, or other caregivers is essential to self-care.*
- *Take regular breaks from caregiving duties by enlisting help from family members or hiring professional caregivers.*
- *Join support groups either online or in person.*
- *Use respite care but remember to get clear on what kind of help is needed first, evaluate potential providers carefully, and do a trial run before fully committing.*
- *Reach out for professional support from counselors or therapists if things become overwhelming.*
- *Patience and understanding are vital when dealing with challenging behavior in dementia patients.*

10

Innovative Approaches & Emerging Treatments

 Dementia may be a cloud but every silver lining has a touch of grey.

— Grateful Dead

The World Health Organization (WHO, 2023) estimates that about 50 million people have some form of dementia, making it a global public health priority requiring urgent attention. Dementia represents a significant global healthcare issue and thus necessitates continued commitment towards research/awareness initiatives to reduce the number of affected individuals.

As you navigate your journey with early-stage dementia, it's understandable to feel uncertain about what lies ahead. But amidst these feelings, there's also reason for optimism. Groundbreaking research is happening worldwide to find better treatments and potentially a cure for this condition.

While there are currently no known cures for most types of dementia, treatments are available that can slow its progression or even reverse some symptoms depending on their cause. The understanding of how lifestyle factors can affect dementia risks is also multiplying.

Now, let's delve into recent advances in medical science that offer hope and new opportunities for those living with early-stage dementia.

Immunotherapy

Research into innovative strategies has grown exponentially over recent years. Among them include immunotherapy-based approaches that target beta-amyloid plaques –protein clumps often found in brains affected by Alzheimer's– and tau tangles –another form of protein associated with this type of dementia– as well as neuroprotective therapies aimed at safeguarding neurons from damage.

Lifestyle and Social Engagement (Non-Drug Treatment)

Moreover, researchers have investigated non-drug treatments such as cognitive training exercises to preserve memory function, physical activity programs, dietary interventions, social engagement activities, music therapy, and art therapy.

For instance, certain studies suggest that high-intensity aerobic exercise could slow down cognitive decline by boosting brain health through improved blood flow and reduced inflammation.

Technology Advances

Another exciting field involves harnessing technology to assist individuals with early-stage dementia in maintaining independence longer. Examples include GPS-enabled devices designed to prevent wandering incidents or apps providing reminders about medication schedules or daily tasks.

Integrative Medicine

In exploring options available now, we must remember integrative approaches combining conventional Western medicine with alternative practices like acupuncture, yoga, or meditation, which have shown benefits when used alongside traditional treatment methods.

Learning about Scientific Works

Scientific research suggests that actively learning about and participating in clinical trials or research studies can profoundly impact your health journey, especially when dealing with a chronic or life-threatening illness.

A study published in the Journal of Clinical Oncology (Niranjan & Wenzei, 2021) found that cancer patients who participated in clinical trials had better outcomes than those who did not. These patients benefit from cutting-edge treatments that are not yet widely available, and medical professionals monitor them throughout the trial.

However, it's important to note that participating in a clinical trial isn't just about potentially receiving new treatments. It's also about contributing to scientific knowledge which could help future patients. As per an article published in The New England Journal of Medicine, individuals participating in clinical trials play a crucial role in advancing medicine and improving healthcare for everyone.

So, there's immense value, personally and societally, when you take an active interest in potential clinical trials or research studies related to your health condition.

When you make decisions based on a thorough understanding of your options (even if it means stepping into unknown territory), you equip yourself with knowledge and power over your health journey. This sense of empowerment may be hard to come by otherwise.

Still, before deciding to participate in any trial or study, consult your healthcare provider first. They can provide valuable insights into whether a particular trial might suit you considering all factors, including potential risks and benefits.

Hope for the Future

> *"Let me say this as clearly as I can: Alzheimer's disease can be prevented, and in many cases, its associated cognitive decline can be reversed. For this is precisely what my colleagues and I have shown in peer-reviewed studies in leading medical journals-studies that, for the first time, describe exactly this remarkable result in patients."*
>
> *- Dr Dale E. Bredesen*

Dr Dale Bredesen, a well-respected neurologist, scientist, and author, conducted extensive research into the causes and potential treatments for Alzheimer's disease. His groundbreaking work suggests that it is possible to slow down the progression of this devastating illness and even reverse its effects (Bredersen, Reversing Cognitive Decline, 2015) .

According to Dr Bredesen's study published in aging, he developed a protocol known as ReCODE (Reversal of Cognitive Decline), which involves personalized lifestyle changes such as diet modifications, regular exercise, quality sleep, and stress management. The results were impressive: out of 10 patients with early Alzheimer's or its precursors who followed his protocol, nine showed significant improvement within six months.

Dr Bredesen doesn't mean that Alzheimer's can be cured overnight or without effort - it requires a comprehensive approach addressing multiple factors simultaneously. However, these findings provide hope where there was little before.

At Macquarie University in Sydney, Australia (Macquarie University , 2020), researchers have discovered a possible treatment tested on mice with late-stage dementia and showing signs it may be able to cure memory loss resulting from Alzheimer's and other forms of dementia. It is early days for the researchers working on further developing gene therapies offering hope to individuals with the disease.

Getting diagnosed with early-stage dementia is daunting but be assured you can use the information and strategies in this book to manage the disease progression and continue to live well.

Stay hopeful as there is more and more research into slowing down and even reversing the effects of this disease. Every day brings us a step closer to unraveling the mysteries behind this complex condition, hoping to ultimately find a cure.

11

Embracing Life Despite Early-Stage Dementia

 Some days there won't be a song in your heart...
Sing anyway!

– Emory Austin

Let me start by saying this: diagnosing early-stage dementia doesn't mean your life is over. It's a severe condition, but it doesn't define you. It's just one part of who you are. And despite this new reality, you can still live a fulfilling and meaningful life.

You may feel overwhelmed or scared right now; that's perfectly normal. But remember, fear only has as much power as we give it. Instead of focusing on the negatives and the unknowns, concentrate on what you can control—your attitude and perspective towards life.

Next comes acceptance. Accepting your diagnosis isn't about giving up; instead, it's about acknowledging the situation so that you can move forward. You'll have good days and bad days—that's okay too!

On those difficult days, don't beat yourself up; instead, be gentle with yourself.

Remember to celebrate your victories—no matter how small they seem—and cherish the moments when things go well. These positive experiences will help keep your spirits high even in challenging times.

Continuing from acceptance is adaptation—the ability to adjust to new situations or changes in your environment becomes crucial at this stage. Simple adjustments like labeling cupboards or setting reminders for tasks can make a big difference in managing day-to-day activities more efficiently.

In 2017, a study published in the Journal of Aging Studies found that individuals diagnosed with early-stage dementia who actively engaged in daily activities reported an increased sense of self-worth and satisfaction compared to those who didn't. So let's call our primary method "The Triple-A Approach"—Attitude, Acceptance & Adaptation—a simple yet effective strategy for embracing life after diagnosis.

Now, let's talk about some potential hurdles along the way.

One common issue many face post-diagnosis is social isolation due to fear or embarrassment about their condition. However, staying connected with friends and family will provide emotional support and help maintain cognitive function longer.

Another potential problem could be dealing with mood swings or depression, which are common symptoms associated with dementia. If these feelings persist or worsen over time, find professional help, such as therapy or counseling services, which offer strategies for coping effectively.

Simple Steps to Embrace Life in Early-Stage Dementia

- Reflect on your attitude towards your diagnosis.
- Practice acceptance daily.
- Start adapting—implement small changes into everyday routines.
- Stay socially active.
- Seek professional help if needed.

You are More than Your Diagnosis: Respect and Advocacy

> *"We need to revolutionize how we think about aging and dementia, so these individuals are recognized as people first."*
> *- Marc Wortmann, Executive Director Alzheimer's Disease International*

It's essential to know that you are entitled to the same respect, dignity, and access to services as anyone else. You can decide about your life and healthcare for as long as possible.

It's essential to understand these rights and how to advocate for them. Advocacy means standing up for your rights and making sure they are respected. It involves expressing your needs clearly and assertively, seeking help, and persisting until you get the support you need.

7 STEPS FOR SUCCESSFUL ADVOCACY

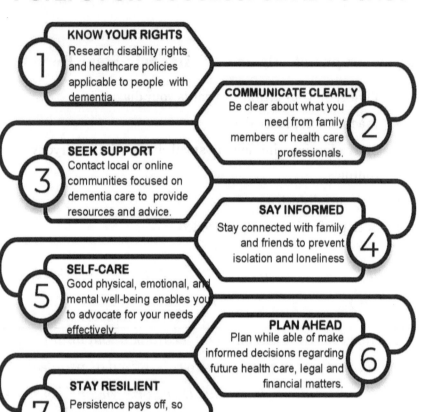

KNOW YOUR RIGHTS
Research disability rights and healthcare policies applicable to people with dementia.

1

COMMUNICATE CLEARLY
Be clear about what you need from family members or health care professionals.

2

SEEK SUPPORT
Contact local or online communities focused on dementia care to provide resources and advice.

3

SAY INFORMED
Stay connected with family and friends to prevent isolation and loneliness

4

SELF-CARE
Good physical, emotional, and mental well-being enables you to advocate for your needs effectively.

5

PLAN AHEAD
Plan while able of make informed decisions regarding future health care, legal and financial matters.

6

STAY RESILIENT
Persistence pays off, so stay resilient even when faced with obstacles.

7

Realistic Future Planning - Don't Give Up Hope

"Never underestimate the power of dreams and influence of the human spirit."

- Wilma Rudolph

Scientific research indicates that early-stage dementia, while challenging, doesn't mean the end of a fulfilling life. Living well in this condition is possible by realistically planning and maintaining hope.

A study published in the Lancet (Gill Livingston, 2020) suggests that individuals diagnosed with early-stage dementia who engage in regular cognitive activities like reading, writing, playing games, or even doing puzzles can slow cognitive decline. Engaging in these activities isn't just about keeping your mind active - it's also about preserving your sense of self and continuing to do things you love.

Moreover, according to experts from the Alzheimer's Association, proactive planning for the future can significantly reduce anxiety associated with dementia. Planning legal and financial affairs and discussing long-term care options in the early stages of dementia gives you more control over decisions affecting your quality of life.

Another crucial aspect is maintaining hope ((Radbourne), Clarke, & Moniz-Cook, 2010). Despite their diagnosis, people living with early-stage dementia who maintain a positive outlook are better able to cope with their situation if they focus on what they can still do rather than what they can't.

Therefore, based on scientific evidence and expert advice, if you or a loved one has been diagnosed with early-stage dementia, keep mentally active through cognitive activities; plan for legal, financial, and long-term care matters; and maintain an optimistic attitude focusing on abilities rather than limitations.

Summing Up

Living with early-stage dementia presents unique challenges, but remember, you can overcome every challenge with persistence and determination, so Don't Give Up!

If things become overwhelming there are numerous resources available, such as social workers specializing in geriatric care management support groups, both offline & online, where individuals share their experiences dealing with similar situations.

But most importantly, remember that while living with dementia has its challenges, *it does not define who you are or what you're capable of achieving (unless you let it).*

Key Takeaways

- *Your Diagnosis Does Not Define You: Remember that there's more to you than just being someone living with dementia—you're still YOU!*
- *Acceptance is Key: Acknowledge your current situation without judgment—it's not about giving up but moving forward positively.*

- *The Power of Adaptation: Small adaptations around the home or work can make day-to-day tasks easier, thus boosting confidence levels significantly.*
- *Social Connectivity Matters: Maintaining solid relationships helps reduce feelings of isolation often associated with dementia while promoting mental health wellness.*
- *Lifestyle changes, including diet modification alongside regular exercise/social engagement, promise to delay onset/disease progression while improving overall quality of life.*
- *Social interactions help keep our brains active, helping fend off symptoms.*
- *Music/art therapy offers therapeutic benefits, enhancing the quality of life while managing symptoms.*
- *Consider utilizing tech aids to enhance daily functioning and reduce caregiver stress levels.*
- *Immunotherapy-based approaches and neuroprotective therapies represent promising avenues for slowing down or halting the progress of early-stage dementia.*
- *Consult your healthcare provider regarding possible inclusion in emerging treatments and trials.*

Conclusion

In travelling through the pages of this book, we have delved deep into the complex world of dementia, particularly its profound impact on many aspects of life. We've explored the challenges, the science, the stories of resilience, and the boundless compassion that caregivers and advocates pour into this cause.

As we conclude our exploration, let us remember that, despite the formidable challenges dementia presents, there is room for hope and progress. The human spirit is indomitable, and science continues to strive for answers and solutions. Together, we can make a difference.

In the face of cognitive decline and its far-reaching effects, we can choose empathy over impatience, understanding over frustration, and love over despair. Our collective awareness and advocacy can dispel the shadows of stigma and fear that have long obscured the lives of those living with dementia.

This book is not just a source of information; it is a call to action.

If you are diagnosed with early-stage dementia, this new understanding empowers you to make a profound impact. You can embrace the challenges, take purposeful steps, and continue living a life that is rich, meaningful, and deeply connected. Your journey is not just about closing a book; it's about opening a new chapter filled with possibilities, compassion, and the unwavering belief that positive change is within your grasp.

As a family member or friend, you are also invited to join a movement of compassion and support for individuals and families affected by dementia; to advocate for more research, better care, and a world that is truly dementia friendly.

Take with you the knowledge that your actions, no matter how small, have the potential to illuminate the path for those touched by dementia. Your kindness and words of encouragement are beacons of hope in the lives of those facing memory loss and the challenges of dementia.

Let this book serve as a guide, a source of inspiration, and a reminder that, even as dementia ebbs and flows, there is room for love, hope, and an unwavering commitment to a better tomorrow. Together, let's rewrite the story of dementia and memory loss, one chapter of understanding and support at a time.

Appendix A: Works Cited

(2012). *World Alzheimer Report 2012 Overcoming the stigma of dementia.* Alzheimers Disease International. Retrieved October 29, 2023, from chrome-extension://efaidnbmnnnibpcajpcglclefindmkaj/https://www.dementia.org.au/sites/default/files/World-Report-2012-summary-EMBARGOED.pdf

(Radbourne), E. L., Clarke, C., & Moniz-Cook, E. (2010). Remaining hopeful in early-stage dementia: A qualitative study. *Aging and Mental Health*, 450-460.

Adam P. Spira, P., Alyssa A. Gamaldo, P., Yang An, M., & al, e. (2013). Self-reported Sleep and β-Amyloid Deposition in Community-Dwelling Older Adults. *JAMA Neurology*, 70(12):1537-1543. doi:10.1001/jamaneurol.2013.4258

Aguirre, E., Hoare, Z., Streater, A., Spector, A., Woods, B., & J Hoe, M. O. (2012). Cognitive stimulation therapy (CST) for people with dementia--who benefits most? *Interational Journal of Geriatric Psychiatry*, 284-290. doi:10.1002/gps.3823

Akhter-Khan, S. C., Tao, Q., Ang, T. F., Itchapurapu, I. S., Alosco, M. L., Mez, J., . . . Qiu, W. Q. (2021). Associations of loneliness with risk of Alzheimer's disease dementia in the Framingham Heart Study. *Alzheimers & Dementia*, 1619-1627. Retrieved from Boston University: https://www.bumc.bu.edu/camed/2021/03/24/midlife-loneliness-is-a-risk-factor-for-dementia-and-alzheimers-disease/#:~:text=Being%20persistently%20lonely%20during%20midlife,who%20have%20never%20felt%20lonely.

Aldridge, H., & Laidlaw, P. F. (2017). Experiences of shame for people with dementia: An Interpretative Phenomenological Analysis. *ResearchGate*. doi:10.1177/1471301217732430

Allen, K. (2021, July 14). *Making Your Home Dementia Friendly.* Retrieved from Bright Focus Foundation: Making Your Home Dementia Friendly

Alzheimer Association. (2021). *2021 Alzheimer's disease facts and figures.* doi: https://doi.org/10.1002/alz.12328

Ashenden, P. (2020, February 18). *Nonverbal Communication: How Body Language & Nonverbal Cues Are Key.* Retrieved from kifesize: https://www.lifesize.com/blog/speaking-without-words/#:~:text=These%20studies%20led%20Dr.,is%20%E2%80%9Cnonverbal%E2%80%9D%20in%20nature.

Bredersen, D. (2015, October 14). Reversing Cognitive Decline. *ntegrative Medicine: A Clinician's Journal (IMCJ)*, 26-29. (C. Gustavson, Interviewer) Retrieved 2023, from https://www.ncbi.nlm.nih.gov/pmc/articles/PMC4712873/

Bredersen, D. (n.d.). *Changing the world of Alzheimer's Disease Research*. Retrieved from Appollo Health: https://www.apollohealthco.com/dr-bredesen/

Broader social interaction keeps older adults more active. (2019, June 1). Retrieved from Harvard Health Publishing: The Journal of Gerontology: Psychological Sciences (2019), social engagement significantly positively affects cognitive functioning among older adults, including those suffering from dementia

Chancellor, B., Duncan, A., & Chatterjee, A. (2014). Art therapy for Alzheimer's disease and other dementias. *Alzheimers Disiease*, 1-11. doi:10.3233/JAD-131295

Collins, R., Anna Hunt, C. Q., Martyr, A., Pentecost, C., & Clare, L. (2022). Methods and approaches for enhancing communication with people with moderate-to-severe dementia that can facilitate their inclusion in research and service evaluation: Findings from the IDEAL programme. *Dementia*. doi:https://doi.org/10.1177/14713012211069449

Communication and Alzheimer's. (n.d.). Retrieved from Alzheimer's Association: https://www.alz.org/help-support/caregiving/daily-care/communications

D.J.Iverson, G.S.Gronseth, M.A.Reger, S.Classen, R.M.Dubinsky, & M.Rizzo. (2010). PracticeParameterupdate:Evaluationand managementofdrivingriskindementia. *American Academy of Neurology*.

Dementia Care: Keeping Loved Ones Safe and Happy at Home. (n.d.). Retrieved from John Hopkins Medicine: https://www.hopkinsmedicine.org/health/wellness-and-prevention/safe-and-happy-at-home

Dieh, J., Mayer, T., Förstl, H., & Kurz, A. (2003). A Support Group for Caregivers of Patients with Frontotemporal Dementia. *Dementia*. doi:https://doi.org/10.1177/1471301203002002002

DiPietro, L. (2001). Physical Activity in Aging: Changes in Patterns and Their Relationship to Health and Function. *Journal of Gerontology*, 13-22.

Duffy, L. M. (1987). Managing urinary incontinence in persons with Alzheimer's disease. *American Journal of Alzheimer's Disease & Other Dementias*. Retrieved from https://journals.sagepub.com/doi/abs/10.1177/153331758700200506?journal Code=ajac

Dufour, A. B., M. L., D'Agata, E. M., D. H., & S. L. (2015). Survival After Suspected Urinary Tract Infection in Individuals with Advanced Dementia. *Journal of the American Geriatrics Society*, 2472-2477. doi:https://doi.org/10.1111/jgs.13833

Fetherstonhaugh, D., Tarziaa, L., & Nay, R. (2012). Being central to decision making means I am still here!:The essence of decision making for people with dementia. *Journal of Aging Studies*, .

Gill Livingston, e. a. (2020). Dementia prevention, intervention, and care: 2020 report of the Lancet Commission. *Lancet*, 396(10248): 413–446.

Gitlin, D. L. (2015, March 5). Behavioral Therapy Helps More Than Drugs For Dementia Patients. (I. Jaffe, Interviewer) NPR. Retrieved from https://www.npr.org/sections/health-shots/2015/03/05/390903112/for-dementia-patients-behavioral-therapy-helps-more-than-drugs

Gitlin, L. N., Winter, L., Burke, J., Chernett, N., Dennis, M. P., & Hauck, W. W. (2008). Tailored Activities to Manage Neuropsychiatric Behaviors in Persons with Dementia and Reduce Caregiver Burden: A Randomized Pilot Study. *Am J Geriatr Psychiatry*, 229-239.

How BBC Two's latest documentary 'Dementia and Us' captured the realities of dementia. (2021). Retrieved from Dementia UK: https://www.dementiauk.org/news/how-bbc-twos-latest-documentary-dementia-and-us-captured-the-realities-of-dementia/

Hurst, J. (n.d.). *Music as a Memory Tool for Patients with Alzheimer's*. Retrieved from Borton University: https://www.bumc.bu.edu/camed/2012/12/12/music-as-a-memory-tool-for-patients-with-alzheimers/

Iaboni, A., Phil, D., & Flint, A. J. (2013). The Complex Interplay of Depression and Falls in Older Adults: A Clinical Review. *American Journal of Geriatric Psychiatry*, 484-492. doi:https://doi.org/10.1016/j.jagp.2013.01.008

Johansson, M., Stomrud, E., Lindberg, O., Westman, E., Johansson, P. M., Westen, D. v., . . . Hansson, O. (2019). Apathy and anxiety are early markers of Alzheimer's disease. *Neurobiology of Aging*, 74-82. doi:https://doi.org/10.1016/j.neurobiolaging.2019.10.008

Jones, R. S., Chow, T., & Gatz, M. (2006). Asian Americans and Alzheimer's disease: Assimilation, culture, and beliefs. *Aging Studies*, 11-25. doi:10.1016/j.jaging.2005.01.001

Lanctôt, K. L., Joan Amatniek, S. A.-I., Arnold, S. E., Ballard, C., Cohen-Mansfield, J., Ismai, Z., . . . Miller, D. S. (2017). Neuropsychiatric signs and symptoms of Alzheimer's disease: New treatment paradigms. *Alzheimers & Dementia*, 440-449.

Legal Planning. (n.d.). Retrieved from Alzheimer's Association: https://www.alz.org/help-support/i-have-alz/plan-for-your-future/legal_planning

Macquarie University . (2020, July 30). *Dementia Researchers Discover World first Gene Therapy that could potentially Reverse Memory Loss from Alzheimer's in Humans.* . Retrieved from The Lighthouse. : https://lighthouse.mq.edu.au/media-relea

Mittelman, M. S., Roth, D. L., Coon, D. W., & Haley, W. E. (2004). Sustained Benefit of Supportive Intervention for Depressive Symptoms in Caregivers of Patients With Alzheimer's Disease. *American JOurnal of Psychiatry*, 850-856.

Moneey Matters MAKING FINANCIAL PLANS AFTER A DIAGNOSIS OF DEMENTIA. (n.d.). Retrieved from Alzheimer's Association: https://alz.org/national/documents/brochure_moneymatters.pdf

Niranjan, S. J., & Wenzei, J. A. (2021). Perceived Institutional Barriers Among Clinical and Research Professionals: Minority Participation in Oncology Clinical Trials. *Journal of Clinical Oncolgy*, 17(5): e666-e675.

Peter H. Van Ness Ph.D., M. a. (2002). Religion, Senescence, and Mental Health: The End of Life Is Not the End of Hope. *American Journal of Geriatric Psychiatry*, 386-397. doi:https://doi.org/10.1097/00019442-200207000-00005

Piersol, C. V., Jensen, L., Lieberman, D., & Arbesman, M. (2018). Occupational Therapy Interventions for People With Alzheimer's Disease. *The American Journal of Occupational Therap.* doi:https://doi.org/10.5014/ajot.2018.721001

Planning After a Dementia Diagnosis. (n.d.). Retrieved from Alzheimer's.gov: https://www.alzheimers.gov/life-with-dementia/planning-for-future

Planning Ahead for Legal Matters. (n.d.). Retrieved from Alzheimer's Association: https://www.alz.org/help-support/caregiving/financial-legal-planning/planning-ahead-for-legal-matters#:~:text=Legal%20planning%20should%20include%3A%201%20Preparing%20for%20long-term,decisions%20on%20behalf%20of%20the%20person%20with%20dementia.

Positive thinking: Stop negative self-talk to reduce stress. (n.d.). Retrieved from Mayo Clinic: https://www.mayoclinic.org/healthy-lifestyle/stress-management/in-depth/positive-thinking/art-20043950

Richardson, N. (2003). Effects of animal-assisted therapy on agitated behaviors and social interactions of older adults with dementia. *Alzheimer's Disease and Other Denetias.* doi:https://doi.org/10.1177/1533317503018006

Sadlon, A., Ensslin, A., Freystätter, G., Gagesch, M., & Heike A Bischoff-Ferrari. (2020). Are patients with cognitive impairment fit to fly? Current evidence and practical recommendations . *Journal of Travel Medicine.*

Sadowsky, C., & Galvin, J. (2012). *Guidelines for the Management of Cognitive and Behavioral Problems in Dementia*. The Journal of the American Board of Family Medicine. Retrieved from https://www.jabfm.org/content/25/3/350.short

Schulz, R., & Sherwood, P. R. (2008). Physical and Mental Health Effects of Family Caregiving. *American Journal of Nursing*.

See, R. S., Thomas, F., Russell, S., Quigley, R., Esterman, A., & Harris, L. (2023). Potentially modifiable dementia risk factors in all Australians and within population groups: an analysis using cross-sectional survey data. *The Lancet*, 717-725. doi:https://doi.org/10.1016/S2468-2667(23)00146-9

Shaw, W. S., T. L., Ziegler, M. G., Dimsdale, J. E., Semple, S. J., & Grant, I. (1999). Accelerated risk of hypertensive blood pressure recordings among alzheimer caregivers. *Journal of Psychosomatic Research*. doi:https://doi.org/10.1016/S0022-3999(98)00084-1

Sheffield, C., Smith, C. A., & Becker, M. (2013). Evaluation of an Agency-Based Occupational Therapy Intervention to Facilitate Aging in Place. *The Gerontologist*, 907-918. Retrieved from Chava Sheffield, PhD, OTR/L, Charles A. Smith, PhD, Mary Becker, MS, OTR/L

Socially active 60-year-olds face lower dementia risk. (2019, August 5). Retrieved from UCL News: https://www.ucl.ac.uk/news/2019/aug/socially-active-60-year-olds-face-lower-dementia-risk#:~:text=Being%20more%20socially%20active%20in,role%20in%20stavi ng%20off%20dementia.

Sofi, F., Macchi, C., Abbate, R., Gensini, G., & Casini, A. (2010). Effectiveness of the Mediterranean Diet: Can It Help Delay or Prevent Alzheimer's Disease? *Journal of Alzheimer's disease*, 795-801. doi:10.3233/JAD-2010-1418

Tanzi, D. R. (2005, October 15). An Interview with Neurogeneticist Rudolph Tanzi. (B. Lom, Interviewer) Retrieved from https://www.ncbi.nlm.nih.gov/pmc/articles/PMC3592619/

Tyndall, A. V., Clark, C. M., Anderson, T. J., Hogan, D. B., Hill, M. D., Longman, R., & Poulin, M. J. (2018). Protective Effects of Exercise on Cognition and Brain Health in Older Adults. *Exercise and Sport Sciences Reviews*, 215-223. Retrieved from https://journals.lww.com/acsm-essr/Fulltext/2018/10000/Protective_Effects_of_Exercise_on_Cognition_an d.4.aspx

Wheeler, M. (2015, February 5). *Forever young: Meditation might slow the age-related loss of gray matter in the brain, say UCLA researchers*. Retrieved from UCLA:

https://newsroom.ucla.edu/releases/forever-young-meditation-might-slow-the-age-related-loss-of-gray-matter-in-the-brain-say-ucla-researchers

WHO. (2023, March 15). *Dementia*. Retrieved from World Health Organization: https://www.who.int/news-room/fact-sheets/detail/dementia/?gclid=CjwKCAjw6eWnBhAKEiwADpnw9loLIZYq-D1U4R3GAmAAAuiOHJDJ2EPUsSdIWvs7gPngVc2ihCH6-hoCxyAQAvD_BwE

Wylie, E. M. (2014). Differing Perspectives on Older Adult Caregiving. *Journal of Applied Gerontology*. doi:https://doi.org/10.1177/0733464813517506

Appendix B: References

Mary Anne Radmacher Quotes & Sayings . (2023, October). Retrieved from search quotes:
https://www.searchquotes.com/quotes/author/Mary_Anne_Radmacher/

Chapter 2: Dementia - Comprehensive Overview
Alzheimer Association. (2021). *2021 Alzheimer's disease facts and figures.* doi:
https://doi.org/10.1002/alz.12328

Alzheimer's Disease Fact Sheet. (n.d.). Retrieved from National Institute on Aging:
https://www.nia.nih.gov/health/alzheimers-disease-fact-sheet

Dementias. (n.d.). Retrieved from Healthy People 2030:
https://health.gov/healthypeople/objectives-and-data/browse-objectives/dementias

Diagnosing dementia. (n.d.). Retrieved from Dementia Australia:
https://www.dementia.org.au/information/diagnosing-dementia

Stages of Alzheimer's & Dementia: Durations & Scales Used to Measure Progression.
(2023, January 26). Retrieved from Dementia Care Central:
https://www.dementiacarecentral.com/aboutdementia/facts/stages/

Understanding Alzheimer's. (n.d.). Retrieved from Bright Focus Foundation:
https://www.brightfocus.org/alzheimers/resources/understanding-alzheimers?gad=1&gclid=CjwKCAjw6eWnBhAKEiwADpnw9ofKlT3KUhHE5D
2VaJno4pWu62zOPU3mvinBIpApUPALlKyrTWEoxBoCXW8QAvD_BwE

Chapter 3: Navigating the Fog
Allen, K. (2021, July 14). *Making Your Home Dementia Friendly.* Retrieved from Bright Focus Foundation: Making Your Home Dementia Friendly

How BBC Two's latest documentary 'Dementia and Us' captured the realities of dementia. (2021). Retrieved from Dementia UK:
https://www.dementiauk.org/news/how-bbc-twos-latest-documentary-dementia-and-us-captured-the-realities-of-dementia/

Staying independent. (n.d.). Retrieved from Alzheimer's Society:
https://www.alzheimers.org.uk/get-support/staying-independent

Chapter 4: Early Onset Dementia Challenges in Younger Adults
If You Have Younger-Onset Alzheimer's Disease. (n.d.). Retrieved from Alzheimer's
Association: https://www.alz.org/help-support/i-have-alz/younger-onset

Shaw, G. (2011, December). *How to Deal with Dementia in the Workplace.* Retrieved
from Brain & Life: https://www.brainandlife.org/articles/how-long-should-
someone-with-dementia-keep-working/

Chapter 5: Lifestyle Changes to Slow Down Progression
Haghighi, A. S. (2022, August 8). *What are the best activities for someone with
dementia?* Retrieved from Medical News Today:
https://www.medicalnewstoday.com/articles/best-activities-for-someone-
with-dementia

Heerema, E. (2021, July 15). *11 Tasty Foods That Reduce Alzheimer's and Dementia
Risk.* Retrieved from very well mind: https://www.verywellhealth.com/foods-
that-reduce-dementia-risk-98464

PHYSICAL ACTIVITIES FOR SENIORS WITH DEMENTIA: 12 EXERCISE IDEAS.
(n.d.). Retrieved from Daily Caring: https://dailycaring.com/12-ideas-for-
exercise-and-physical-activities-for-seniors-with-dementia/

Why Sudoku is the Perfect Brain Exercise for Beginners and Seniors. (2023, June 29).
Retrieved from Ask: https://www.ask.com/culture/sudoku-perfect-brain-
exercise-beginners-
seniors?utm_content=params%3Aad%3DdirN%26qo%3DserpInd

ex%260%3D740004&ueid=1542DD2B-119F-4F9C-ACDF-5DAE2FD6ECCB

Wheeler, M. (2015, February 5). *Forever young: Meditation might slow the age-related
loss of gray matter in the brain, say UCLA researchers.* Retrieved from UCLA:
https://newsroom.ucla.edu/releases/forever-young-meditation-might-slow-
the-age-related-loss-of-gray-matter-in-the-brain-say-ucla-researchers

Reducing Stress. (n.d.). Retrieved from Alzheimer;s Association:
https://www.alz.org/help-support/i-have-alz/live-well/reducing-stress

Berk, L., Warmenhoven, F., Os, J. v., & Boxtel, M. v. (2018). Mindfulness Training for People With Dementia and Their Caregivers: Rationale, Current Research, and Future Directions. *Frontiers in Psychology*. doi:10.3389/fpsyg.2018.00982

Socially active 60-year-olds face lower dementia risk. (2019, August 5). Retrieved from UCL News: https://www.ucl.ac.uk/news/2019/aug/socially-active-60-year-olds-face-lower-dementia-risk#:~:text=Being%20more%20socially%20active%20in,role%20in%20staving%20off%20dementia.

Tips for Daily Life. (n.d.). Retrieved from Alzheimer's Association: https://www.alz.org/help-support/i-have-alz/live-well/tips-for-daily-life

Daily Living. (n.d.). Retrieved from Alzheimer's Society: https://www.alzheimers.org.uk/get-support/daily-living

Chapter 6: Planning for Your Future - Legal, Financial, and Health Considerations

Legal Planning. (n.d.). Retrieved from Alzheimer's Association: https://www.alz.org/help-support/i-have-alz/plan-for-your-future/legal_planning

End-of-Life Planning. (n.d.). Retrieved from Alzheimers Association: https://www.alz.org/help-support/i-have-alz/plan-for-your-future/end_of_life_planning

Moneey Matters MAKING FINANCIAL PLANS AFTER A DIAGNOSIS OF DEMENTIA. (n.d.). Retrieved from Alzheimer's Association: https://alz.org/national/documents/brochure_moneymatters.pdf

Planning After a Dementia Diagnosis. (n.d.). Retrieved from Alzheimer's.gov: https://www.alzheimers.gov/life-with-dementia/planning-for-future

Planning Ahead for Legal Matters. (n.d.). Retrieved from Alzheimer's Association: https://www.alz.org/help-support/caregiving/financial-legal-planning/planning-ahead-for-legal-matters#:~:text=Legal%20planning%20should%20include%3A%201%20Preparing%20for%20long-term,decisions%20on%20behalf%20of%20the%20person%20with%20dementia.

Chapter 7: Navigating Relationships & Emotional Support

Telling people about your dementia diagnosis. (n.d.). Retrieved from Alzheimer's Society: https://www.alzheimers.org.uk/get-support/daily-living/telling-people-about-your-dementia-diagnosis

When to go public with a dementia diagnosis. (2019, March 7). Retrieved from Hella Health: https://www.hellahealth.com/blog/wellness/when-to-tell-you-have-dementia/

Chapter 8: Navigating the Healthcare Maze

Building a Care Team. (n.d.). Retrieved from Alzheimer's Association: https://www.alz.org/help-support/i-have-alz/plan-for-your-future/building_a_care_team

Care homes: When is the right time and who decides? (n.d.). Retrieved from Alzheimer's Society: https://www.alzheimers.org.uk/get-support/help-dementia-care/care-homes-who-decides-when

Morris, S. Y. (2023, July 27). *Dementia and Incontinence: Is There a Link?* Retrieved from healthline: https://www.healthline.com/health/dementia/incontinence-care

The Link Between UTI and Dementia in Older Adults. (n.d.). Retrieved from Pathways: https://pathwayshealth.org/link-uti-dementia-older-adults/#:~:text=According%20to%20Alzheimers.net%2C%20if%20a%20senior%20patient%20already,elderly%20patients%20may%20not%20complain%20of%20such%20pain.

Urinary tract infections and dementia. (n.d.). Retrieved from Alzheimer's Society: https://www.alzheimers.org.uk/get-support/daily-living/urinary-tract-infections-utis-dementia

Chapter 9: The Essential Caregiver's Guide

Carers: looking after yourself. (n.d.). Retrieved from Alzheimer's Society: https://www.alzheimers.org.uk/get-support/help-dementia-care/looking-after-yourself

Tips for Caregivers and Families of People With Dementia. (n.d.). Retrieved from Alzheimers.gov: https://www.alzheimers.gov/life-with-dementia/tips-caregivers

Chapter 10: Innovative Approaches & Emerging Treatments

Bredersen, D. (2015, October 14). Reversing Cognitive Decline. *ntegrative Medicine: A Clinician's Journal (IMCJ)*, 26-29. (C. Gustavson, Interviewer) Retrieved 2023, from https://www.ncbi.nlm.nih.gov/pmc/articles/PMC4712873/

Bredersen, D. (n.d.). *Changing the world of Alzheimer's Disease Research*. Retrieved from Appollo Health: https://www.apollohealthco.com/dr-bredesen/

D. Bredesen, Amos, e., L Canick, Raji, M. A., Fiala, M., & Ahdidan, J. (2016). Reversal of cognitive decline in Alzheimer's disease. . *Aging*, 8(6), 1250-1258. doi:https://doi.org/10.18632/aging.100981

The future of vaccines for Alzheimer's and dementia. (2023, June 29). Retrieved from Alzheimers Disease International: https://www.alzint.org/resource/the-future-of-vaccines-for-alzheimers-and-dementia/

Chapter 11: Embracing Life Despite a Diagnosis

Live Well Online Resources. (n.d.). Retrieved from Alzheimer's Association: https://www.alz.org/help-support/i-have-alz/live-well/live_well_online_resources

The global voice on dementia. (n.d.). Retrieved from Alzheimer's Disease International: https://www.alzint.org/

Appendix C: Suggested Reading and Information

Early Onset Alzheimer's

* ❖ What I Wish People Knew About Dementia: From Someone Who Knows – Wendy Mitchell
* ❖ I Wish I Had a Clue About Early-Onset Dementia - Edna Hawes

Recognising Dementia in Loved Ones

* ❖ Does My Mom Have Dementia? How to Recognize and Deal with Dementia in Your Loved Ones – Erik Lande, Robert Duff

Information for Caregivers

* ❖ Dementia Behaviors - Caregivers Survival Guide: Simple, Proven Methods to Control and Defuse the Situation Before it Blows up! – Grace Southerly
* ❖ Day to Day: Living With Dementia: A Mayo Clinic Guide for Offering Care and Support – Angela M. Lunde
* ❖ Loving Someone Who Has Dementia: How to Find Hope while Coping with Stress and Grief – Pauline Boss
* ❖ The 36-Hour Day: A Family Guide to Caring for People Who Have Alzheimer's Disease and Other Dementias - Nancy L Mace, Peter V Rabins
* ❖ Chicken Soup for the Soul: Living with Alzheimer's and Other Dementias: 101 Stories of Caregiving, Coping, and Compassion – Amy Newmark, Angela Timashenka Geiger

Advocacy and Rights

* ❖ How We Think About Dementia: Personhood, Rights, Ethics, the Arts and What They Mean for Care – Julin C. Hughes

Activity Books

* ❖ Word Search for Seniors Large Print: 200 Word Search Puzzles with Solutions - Large Print – Bernstein
* ❖ Fun and Relaxing Activities for Adults: Puzzles for People with Dementia [Large-Print]: 1 – Might Oak Books

- ❖ Memory Activities Book for Seniors: 7 Tested Solutions to Strengthen Your Memory Quickly and Easily Using the Montessori Method. Also Useful for Alzheimer's, Post Stroke, and Dementia – Michel Brain
- ❖ Exercise Your Brain: Brain Exercises For Dementia - Brain Training Activities For Seniors And Dementia – Danielle Grimaldi

Lifestyle

- ❖ Dementia Diet Cookbook: Healthy Memory Improvement Meal Recipe to Manage Alzheimer's and Improve Thinking – Jonson Mayour
- ❖ Brain-Boosting Diet Cookbook for Seniors: The 20 Nutrient-Rich Recipes for a Sharp Mind and Preventing Dementia – William B. Gomes
- ❖ ALZHEIMER'S DIET COOKBOOK FOR SENIORS: 30 Quick, Easy and Delicious Brain-friendly Recipes to Prevent Dementia and Cognitive Decline – Brenda Harris
- ❖ CHAIR YOGA: A GENTLE PRACTICE FOR SENIORS SEEKING TO ENHANCE WELLBEING: Relieve Pain and Stiffness with Gentle, Seated Yoga Poses – Justin J Williams
- ❖ Balance Exercise for Seniors 50, 60 and Beyond: Live Without Fear of Falling: 50 Videos, 30 Chair and 20 bodyweight exercises + 8 Week Workouts to Improve... Posture and Boost Self-Confidence. – David O'Connor
- ❖ Stretching Exercises for Seniors Over 60: A Safe and Effective Way to Improve Your Health, Flexibility and Mobility – Gloria N. Rubin
- ❖ Strength Training for Seniors Over 70 – Trainer Theo

Index

A

acceptance, 10, 32, 36, 118, 166

acetylcholinesterase inhibitors. *See medication*

acknowledging your feelings, 34

acupuncture, 162

adult daycare. *See respite care*

advocacy and rights, 156, 168

aerobic exercise, 68

affirmations, 76

agitation, 22, 37

Alzheimer's disease. *See* types of dementia

anticipatory grief, 125

antioxidants that help prevent damage to brain cells, 66

anxiety, 22, 23, 33, 37, 48, 52, 70, 75, 77, 81, 125, 132, 141, 142, 145

ApoE4. *See* risk genes

art therapy, 77

assisted living. *See* care options, *See* care options

automated medication dispenser, 49

B

balance activities, 68

balancing safety with independence, 124

behavior changes, 14, 22, 58

beta-amyloid deposition. *See* sleep hygiene

beta-amyloid plaques, 161

brain healthy lifestyle: exercise, 17

breathing exercises, 73

burnout, 140, 142, 145

C

card matching. *See memory games*

care options: home care; assisted living, 86, 97, 170

care plan, 36, 80, 128

caregiver, 139

caregiver self-care, 140

caregiver self-care, 142

CBT. *See* Cognitive Behavioral Therapy, *See* Cognitive Behavioral Therapy, *See* Cognitive Behavioral Therapy

changes in personality, 14

choosing the right healthcare provider, 129

clinical trials, 162

Cognitive Behavioral Therapy, 118; CBT, 33

cognitive decline, 8, 19, 21, 25, 43, 50, 119

cognitive stimulation activities: puzzles; memory games, 36, 65, 70, 71

cognitive stimulation therapy: CST, 35

complications, 26